The
KAYAKING
SOURCEBOOK

· ·

Help Us Keep This Book Up to Date

Every effort has been made by the author and editors to make this book as accurate and useful as possible. However, many things can change after a book is published—organizations close, phone numbers change, companies come under new management, etc.

We would love to hear from you concerning your experiences with this sourcebook and how you feel it could be made better and be kept up to date. While we may not be able to respond to all comments and suggestions, we'll take them to heart and we'll also make certain to share them with the author. Please send your comments and suggestions to the following address:

The Globe Pequot Press
Reader Response/Editorial Department
P.O. Box 833
Old Saybrook, CT 06475

Or you may E-mail us at:

editorial@globe-pequot.com

Thanks for your input, and happy paddling!

THE KAYAKING SOURCEBOOK

A COMPLETE RESOURCE FOR GREAT KAYAKING ON RIVERS, LAKES, AND THE OPEN SEA

by

Cecil Kuhne

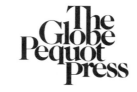

The Globe Pequot Press

Old Saybrook, Connecticut

To the editors of *Canoe & Kayak* magazine

Editor: Don Graydon
Illustrations by Lisa Reneson
Cover photo by Julie Bidwell. Equipment used in front cover photo courtesy North Cove Outfitters, 75 Main Street, Old Saybrook, Connecticut 06475; (860) 388–6585.
Product photos courtesy: Ainsworth, Betsie Bay Kayak, Cricket Designs, Current Designs/We-no-nah Canoe, Dagger Canoe Co., Eddyline, Feathercraft, Grey Owl Paddles, Karel's Fiberglass Products, Kayak Lab, Kotatat, Kruger Canoes, Lotus Designs, Morley's Cedar Canoe, Nimbus Paddles, Northwest River Supplies, Old Town Canoe Co., Pacific Canoe Base, Perception Inc., Prijon/Wildwasser Sport USA, Pygmy Boats, Inc., Sawyer Paddles & Oars, Sea Bright Kayak, Seavivor, Stearns, Inc., Superior Kayaks, Venturesport, Inc., Walden Paddlers, Inc., Werner Paddles, Wilderness Systems, Woodstrip Watercraft

Library of Congress Cataloging-in-Publication Data is available.

ISBN 0-7627-0189-7

Manufactured in the United States of America
First Edition/First Printing

Contents

Preface

My first brush with kayaking occurred back in 1972, when I read an account of a middle-aged physician from Salmon, Idaho, named Walt Blackadar who had just returned from paddling the dreaded Turnback Canyon on Alaska's Alsek River. Blackadar had somehow survived the ordeal of treacherous rapids, frigid waters, and aggressive grizzlies. That same summer the television was filled with coverage of the kayak slalom events at the Olympic Games in Munich. The images of Blackadar and of Munich captured my imagination, and I was obsessed to find out more.

The only book I could find on the subject was Peter Whitney's *Whitewater Sport,* a thin volume with simplistic prose and crude stick-figure drawings. I pored over the book and a black-and-white equipment catalog that showed a few generic fiberglass kayaks, a couple of do-it-yourself spray skirt kits, and some thick scuba-diving wet suits. Little did I imagine then that twenty-five years later I'd still be poring over kayaking books and catalogs—only now they're a lot more sophisticated. And since that Olympic summer I've had the great fortune to paddle waters on every continent except Antarctica.

In the past decade few outdoor pursuits have captured the attention of the American public more than kayaking. The kayak, it seems, is the ideal craft in which to pierce deep into the backcountry via its lakes and rivers and to explore isolated ocean coasts. It is light, it is sleek, and most of all, it is fast. On closer view, there are more aspects to this endeavor than you might imagine. There is casual touring, with its relaxed pace and its access to picturesque coves and alpine lakes. There is sea kayaking, with its share of adventure on unpredictable ocean swells and long coastal journeys. There is whitewater kayaking, with adrenaline-pumping fervor on rivers that drop suddenly from sight into a confusion of foam and fury. There is also playboating, where the focus is on tricky maneuvers in the river's currents. And then there is surf kayaking, where you can spend countless hours paddling in and out of the ocean's waves.

To satisfy these various interests, there are now some seventy kayak manufacturers who produce hundreds of designs, in an array of sophisticated materials, to meet almost any conceivable need. Kayaking is both a broad and a specialized subject—which renders it a fascinating one. A sourcebook can touch only highlights of this magnificent pastime, and the format of this book is a simple one. The first four chapters will introduce you to the basics of kayak design and materials and to the essentials of paddling technique. Then we'll go into more detail about the main categories of paddling and types of kayaks, with chapters on casual touring boats, sea kayaks, whitewater kayaks, whitewater playboats, surf kayaks, sit-on-top designs, folding kayaks, and inflatables. There also is a chapter on build-your-own boats. In each of these chapters, we'll present information on many of the models currently on the market, as well as books and videos on skills and technique. A separate chapter will cover the myriad paddling accessories—life jackets, spray skirts, helmets, flotation, and so on—that you'll need to be comfortable and secure on the water. And lastly, we'll discuss kayak safety and rescue. Throughout the book, you'll be introduced to the companies and to the individuals who give form and character to this glorious sport.

The main purpose of this sourcebook is to acquaint you with manufacturers, books, videos, and other resources so that you can dig a little deeper on your own. Along the way we hope you'll be entertained—and yes, even inspired—by the advice and trip accounts that are liberally scattered throughout.

There is one caveat, however (isn't there always?). This book is not intended as a substitute

The Lure of Touring

"Comfortably seated in your silent, swift kayak, you become a participant in a natural world unfortunately abandoned by all too many of us. You set your own pace, your own goals: you may enjoy an hour-long cruise along the beach or you may embark on a month-long voyage through these north Pacific islands—or along the Maine coast, through the Florida Keys, or from island to island along the north coast of Lake Superior. You may use your boat for exercise, or as a platform for fishing or birdwatching. It may become your vantage point for photography or painting. All those 'mays' are at your paddle tips. The truth is that all your voyages will lead back inside yourself, and along the way you'll meet yourself again."

—Dennis Stuhaug
Kayaking Made Easy

for the real thing; in other words, vicarious experiences don't count. So grab a kayak, arm yourself with all the knowledge you can glean from the experts, and then go forth into this great big beautiful world of paddling. Like they say: life is short, paddle hard!

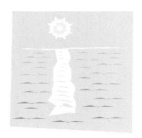

Chapter 1
The Kayak: An Introduction

Over the centuries, the earliest known inhabitants of the Arctic regions of North America developed a remarkable paddle-powered craft for traveling over icy bays, inlets, and even the open ocean. These light and fast-moving boats were designed primarily for hunting and fishing.

Called kayaks by the Eskimos, these decked, single-cockpit boats were masterpieces of primitive engineering. Made of driftwood and the skins and sinews of animals, the ancient Eskimo kayak was a remarkably resilient and durable craft, both light to handle and swift in the water.

As early as the sixteenth century, English explorers in the northern seas saw Eskimos using kayaks to travel and hunt on the water. In 1865 Londoner John MacGregor built his famous *Rob Roy* kayak and toured many of Europe's rivers in it. He called the decked boat a canoe, and his book about his travels, *A Thousand Miles in the Rob Roy Canoe on Rivers and Lakes of Europe*, was an instant best seller, and thereby popularized the sport.

The recommended resource for kayak history is *The Bark Canoes and Skin Boats of North America*, by Edwin Tappan Adney and Howard I. Chapelle (Washington, D.C.: Smithsonian Institute Press, reprint edition, 1983).

George Dyson has done a magnificent job of tracing the story of the baidarka in his lavishly illustrated book *Baidarka: The Kayak* (Seattle: Alaska Northwest Books, 1986). Also of interest is *The Aleutian Kayak*, by Wolfgang Brinck (Camden, Maine: Ragged Mountain Press, 1995). The Baidarka Historical Society works to preserve knowledge of this fascinating boat. (The society can be contacted at P.O. Box 5454, Bellingham, WA 98227.)

The Modern Kayak

Not long ago, a kayak was just a kayak. There was essentially one multipurpose design that could be paddled everywhere—across a lake one day and down a

1

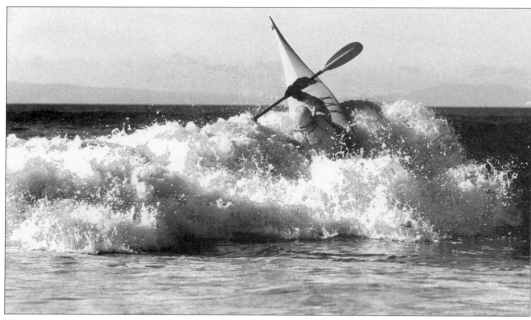

Kayaking can be an adventure (courtesy Current Designs)

whitewater river the next. Like most compromises, it did a lot of things well, but none of them *really* well. Similar boats are still being built today, but more models are designed for specific uses—for speed, the sea, whitewater, playing on waves, or perhaps just a gentle afternoon cruise across a lake.

To understand the differences among kayaks, let's divide them into categories: casual touring boats (recreational kayaks), sea kayaks (also called touring kayaks), whitewater kayaks, whitewater playboats, surf kayaks, sit-on-tops, folding kayaks, and inflatables. As you can see, there is no shortage of options, which of course com-

Kayaks Down the Nile

As a boy of fifteen, John Goddard prepared a list of 127 life goals. He accomplished all but a few of them, including explorations of the Nile, Amazon, and Congo Rivers. Goddard, now in his 70s, is credited with being the first person to explore the entire length of both the Nile and Congo Rivers. In 1950 he set off with two French companions to paddle the length of the Nile—4,145 miles—by kayak.

During the nine-month adventure, they were attacked by hippos and wild dogs, nearly drowned in rapids, shot at by Egyptian river pirates, almost buried alive in a blinding sandstorm, stoned by a mob of hostile Arabs, and struck with malaria and dysentery. The saga is well chronicled in Goddard's book *Kayaks Down the Nile* (Provo, Utah: Brigham Young University Press, 1979), long out of print but worth seeking out.

plicates the decision of which boat to choose for your own kayaking. And virtually every kind of kayak has been designed for tandem as well as solo use.

Following is a brief description of each type of kayak. In the next chapter, we'll discuss basic design features and how they affect performance in order to help you decide just which kayak is right for you.

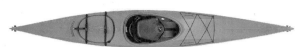

Perception's Spectrum

Dagger Canoe's Frolic

Casual Touring Boats (Recreational Kayaks)

Casual touring boats are all-around designs meant for mild river trips, weekend ventures on sheltered waters, and other low-key touring uses. These recreational boats are easier to turn than the sea kayaks used for serious touring, but do not *track* (maintain travel in a straight line) as well.

Sea Kayaks (Touring Kayaks)

Sea kayaks are designed for extended trips and all the gear they entail. They will handle a generous load at a fair rate of speed under conditions you'll find on oceans, bays, lakes, and big rivers. Though these boats are often called sea kayaks, they're certainly not restricted to the ocean, and they are also widely termed touring kayaks. These long kayaks are very stable and track well, but they don't turn as easily as the somewhat shorter boats used for casual touring.

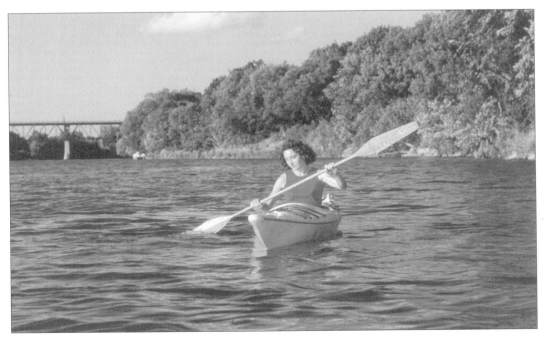

Kayaking can be contemplative (courtesy Grey Owl Paddles)

Canoe or Kayak?

Americans share a common language with the British—or so it seems. We call decked boats kayaks, and we call open boats canoes. The British, on the other hand, refer to all of these boats as canoes—even the ones we call kayaks. But at least they concede there's a difference: They call the real canoe a Canadian canoe.

Whitewater Kayaks

Whitewater kayaks offer exceptional maneuverability in the rigorous environment of a rapids-studded river. These kayaks are short, with round bottoms and a high degree of upturn in the ends (called *rocker*), making them easy to turn. These same characteristics make then unsuitable for a long trip because it's difficult to paddle them in a straight line.

Whitewater Playboats

Extreme versions of whitewater kayaks are called playboats, made for agility in cavorting on a river's waves and currents. Squirt boats, a variant of the playboat, can even negotiate the currents under the surface.

Surf Kayaks

Surf kayaks—often called surf skis and wave skis—are designed for riding the waves of the ocean. Wave skis, short and featuring a blunt nose, are derived from surfboards. Surf skis are much longer and resemble a sea kayak in design.

Sit-on-top Kayaks

Most kayaks have a hull in which the paddler sits—but increasingly popular are the sit-on-top kayaks, designed to be sat upon rather than in. Sit-on-tops come in al-

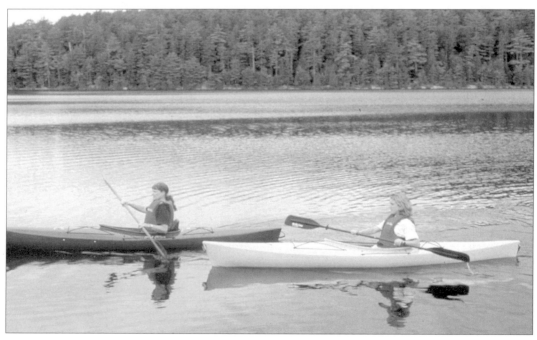

Loon 120 (courtesy Old Town Canoe Co.)

Zen and the Art of Paddling

It's not your typical kayak book, but *The Starship and the Canoe*, by Kenneth Brower (New York: Holt, Rinehart, 1973), is the true story of an eccentric visionary who builds gigantic kayaks to cruise the Pacific Northwest seas and of his astrophysicist father, who dreams of building a nuclear-powered spaceship the size of Chicago. The kayak involved is the resurrection of the Aleut kayak that Russian fur hunters named the baidarka. This is the compelling story of two men, two arks, and two views of man's destiny.

most as many shapes and styles as the more traditional kayaks, and can be put to a variety of uses depending on the particular design.

Folding Kayaks

Folding kayaks are made of fabric stretched tightly across a collapsible metal or wooden frame. Because they fold down, they are relatively easy to store and to transport in cars, trains, or planes. Depending on design, they can be used for many kinds of kayak travel.

Inflatable Kayaks

Inflatables have become practical and efficient alternatives to hard-shell kayaks for some uses, especially in whitewater. An inflatable provides great buoyancy but lacks some of the maneuverability of a traditional hard-shell. With self-bailing floors and high-tech fabrics and coatings, the design of inflatable kayaks has blossomed since their introduction in the 1960s, and some of the models are approaching the performance levels of their more rigid brethren.

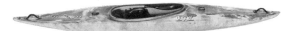

Dagger Canoe Co.'s Blast

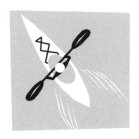

Chapter 2
Choosing a Kayak

Choosing a kayak involves an understanding of the principles of kayak design and construction and the impact they have on the performance of a boat. Once you understand these basics, you can explore the different types of boats on the market. You'll get the details on manufacturers and the models they build in later chapters discussing each type of kayak.

Kayak Design

Nine design features can greatly affect a boat's performance: length, width, keel shape (also known as rocker), bottom shape, side shape, chine shape, bow shape, volume, and cockpit size. Let's look at each.

Length

More than any other single factor, the length of a kayak determines how the boat will handle. The boat's maneuverability, its stability, and its ability to travel in a straight line (called tracking) are affected by length. At the short end of the range are playboats

at 9 or 10 feet; in the middle are whitewater and casual touring boats which are usually 13 or 14 feet; and at the long end of the spectrum are sea kayaks and surf kayaks extending from 17 to 22 feet (or more).

A long casual touring kayak or sea kayak offers a number of performance advantages. It is more stable and more spacious than a shorter model. In addition, it is easier to paddle because it tracks better. This allows you to worry less about the boat veering from side to side and to focus instead on making the boat go faster.

In heavy waves, a longer boat tends to give you a smoother ride because it isn't being tossed to and fro as easily as a smaller boat would be. Of course, if a long boat happens to straddle the crests of the waves, it might provide a rougher ride than a shorter boat that fits nicely between the waves, going up one side and down the other.

For whitewater use, a shorter kayak is a necessity, and the trend in recent years has been toward amazingly shorter designs. The

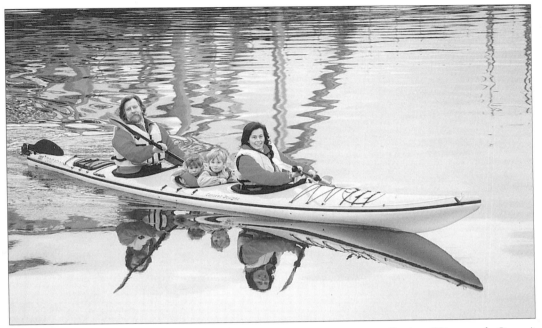

Family kayaking calls for the right-sized boat (courtesy Current Designs/We-no-nah Canoe)

greatest advantage of a short boat is its ability to make quick turns or spins, a characteristic that is helpful on rock-studded rivers where a lot of maneuvering is required.

Width

A kayak's stability is largely determined by its width. Generally, the wider the boat, the more stable it will be. Unfortunately, a wider boat is not as responsive to a paddle stroke simply because the boat has more surface area in the water. Most casual touring boats are wider (and therefore more stable) than sea kayaks, which tend to be narrower so that the boat will glide faster through the water. Most whitewater kayaks and playboats are wide, so that the boats are less likely to be flipped over by the violent action of rapids.

Keel Shape (Rocker)

The uplift at each of a kayak's ends is called *rocker*, and it influences a boat's maneuverability as well as how easy it is to paddle the boat in a straight line. Kayaks that are more upturned in the ends have less surface in the water and therefore pivot more easily. Kayaks with less upturn tend to travel in a straight line more easily. Most whitewater boats and playboats have generous rocker, while most casual touring boats and sea kayaks do not.

Bottom Shape

The bottom of a kayak can range from flat to moderately curved to heavily curved to V-shaped. Bottom shape will determine the boat's stability, maneuverability, and tracking.

A flat-bottomed kayak will be very stable at first (known as initial stability), but

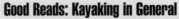
Good Reads: Kayaking in General

Here are some good general introductory books on kayaking. Check the individual chapters on each type of kayaking for lists of books about those specialties.

Kayaking: Whitewater and Touring Basics, by Steven M. Krauzer (New York: W. W. Norton, 1995): one of the best all-around books on kayaking; nicely photographed and illustrated.

Kayaking Made Easy, by Dennis Stuhaug (Old Saybrook, Connecticut: The Globe Pequot Press, 1998): the favored beginning primer for casual touring.

The Complete Book of Sea Kayaking, by Derek C. Hutchinson (Old Saybrook, Connecticut: The Globe Pequot Press, 1995): a well-written guide to sea kayaking, now in its fourth edition.

Kayaking: Whitewater and Sea, by Kent Ford (Human Kinetics, 1995): a basic guide to whitewater boating and to touring, by one of the sport's most renowned practitioners.

as it begins to turn on its side, it will quickly become unstable. A more rounded hull has poor initial stability, but as the boat begins to tip over, it can easily be stabilized (known secondary stability) by an experienced boater. Neither a flat-bottomed nor a rounded-hull boat has especially great tracking ability, which is better provided by a V-shaped hull.

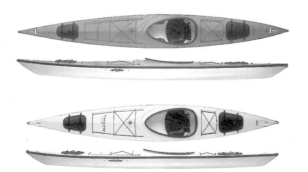

Same boat, different size, different uses: The Merlin XT offers high volume and good stability, suitable for serious touring. The shorter, sporty version, the Merlin LT, is a low-volume kayak best for day trips. (courtesy Eddyline)

Most casual touring boats have a flatter bottom (for stability), most whitewater boats have a rounded bottom (for easier righting), and most sea kayaks have a V-shaped or arch-shaped bottom (for better tracking).

Side Shape

The side shape of many kayaks, as viewed from the end, is flared—angling outward from the waterline up to the top edge (the gunwale). Others have straight sides that rise vertically from the water. Still other kayaks have tumblehome sides, which curve inward toward the gunwale.

Hulls with greater flare have better initial stability. But boats with straight or tumblehome sides have better secondary stability, making them more nimble and easier to roll back up after tipping.

Chine Shape

The area where the bottom of the kayak meets its sides is called the chine. If

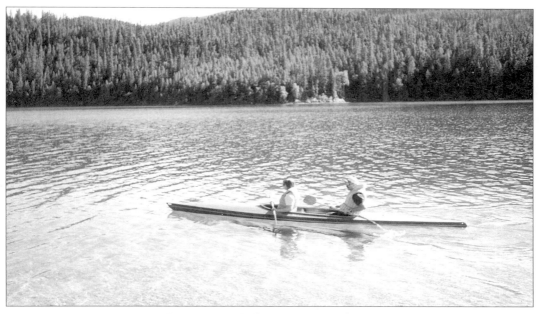

Choosing wood: the 20' TK2 kayak (courtesy Morley's Cedar Canoe)

the angle between the two approaches a sharp, right angle, it is called a hard chine. If it is a rounded angle, it is called a soft chine. A hard chine—usually combined with a flat bottom—provides great initial stability but poor secondary stability as the boat is leaned. A soft chine—usually combined with a more rounded bottom—provides poor initial stability but good secondary stability in the hands of an experienced boater.

Most casual touring boats have a hard chine (for good initial stability), while most whitewater boats have a soft chine (for easier righting). Sea kayaks are usually somewhere in between.

Bow Shape

Sea kayaks typically have narrow, pointed bows that easily cut through the water for faster passage. A broader bow, found in most whitewater kayaks, will not be as efficient but will have more buoyancy,

which is useful in negotiating rapids. Casual touring boats have an in-between shape, with a more blunt bow that is useful for storing gear.

Volume

The volume of a boat is literally the amount of its interior space. In whitewater boats this is important, because volume provides buoyancy. In casual touring boats and sea kayaks, volume determines the amount of gear you can take along. Regardless of its design, a larger boat is less maneuverable, but the added volume makes the boat more comfortable because it affords more space for your legs and feet.

Cockpit Size

The size of the cockpit opening determines the ease with which you can enter and exit the boat. A smaller cockpit allows a snugger fit, making it somewhat easier for

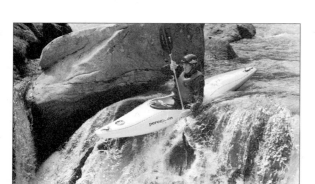

Whitewater action in an Overflow X white-water kayak (courtesy Perception)

the paddler to roll the boat back up after tipping.

Kayak Materials

Kayaks can be built from polyethylene plastic, fiberglass, composite materials, wood, and canvas. Each type of material has a different weight. A lighter boat is easier to handle, both in and out of the water. But to ensure that lightweight kayaks are strong, they must be made of durable (and expensive) materials.

Most casual touring boats, whitewater boats, and playboats are made of plastic. Many sea kayaks are also made of plastic, but a number are still made of fiberglass or other composite material.

Gear Update

The specifications of all kayaks on the market and their related gear can be found in the annual buyers' guide of *Canoe & Kayak* magazine, published in every December issue. It's an invaluable resource for gear-obsessed paddlers of all types.

Plastic

The biggest advantage of polyethylene in kayak manufacturing is its low cost and its ability to be molded and mass produced. It is also very durable, which is especially important in situations where a boat will take a beating on rocks or in heavy waves.

There are two basic types of polyethylene—linear and cross-linked. Both are durable, but cross-linked polyethylene is somewhat stiffer. Linear polyethylene, on the other hand, can be recycled, while cross-linked cannot.

Likewise, there are two types of molding—roto-molding and blow-molding. The main difference in the finished product is that a blow-molded boat is stiffer (and heavier).

Roto-molding is the most common manufacturing method. In it, powdered polyethylene is poured into a heated mold that is rotated until the mold is completely coated with a layer of plastic. The mold cools and is opened to reveal a boat. The

Epic, a roto-molded kayak by Wilderness Systems

whole process takes about an hour.

Blow-molding uses extreme pressure to melt plastic pellets and force the molten plastic into molds, where it remains until it cools. The blow-molding process is fast, taking about ten minutes to form a boat.

Composites

Composite kayaks may be made with fiberglass, with Kevlar (which is more durable, lighter in weight, and more expensive than fiberglass), or with one of many proprietary formulas, developed by individual manufacturers, that combine various fibers and resins. In general, composite boats are made with layers of synthetic fabric placed into a mold and then covered with a resin that hardens the fabric into the shape of a boat.

Very few whitewater boats are now made of composites because these materials cannot take the beating of rocks and rapids that polyethylene can. Some sea kayaks are made of fiberglass or Kevlar because these materials provide a lighter boat than polyethylene and because the shapes of boats produced from these composites seem to have a finer definition than is currently possible with polyethylene. Most casual touring boats are made of polyethylene simply because it is less expensive.

Wood

Kayaks can be made of wood—either long, thin planks or larger pieces of plywood. After the hull of a wooden kayak is constructed, it is typically lined with fiberglass cloth and resin for waterproofing and durability. These boats are beautiful to behold and very lightweight, but they are less durable and require more maintenance than synthetic boats.

Fabric

Folding kayaks are made of an outer skin of coated nylon or canvas fabric, which is stretched tightly over a collapsible wood or aluminum frame. These boats have been around almost a hundred years, and their devotees find them the perfect compromise of handling and portability. While not as durable as most hardshell boats (especially in heavy whitewater), the

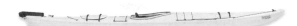

Sea Lion S, a composite kayak by Perception

high-quality models are amazingly resilient.

Kayaks and Compromise

As you begin looking for a kayak that meets your particular needs, keep firmly in mind that any boat design is a compromise of factors that determine tracking (the ability to travel in a straight line), speed,

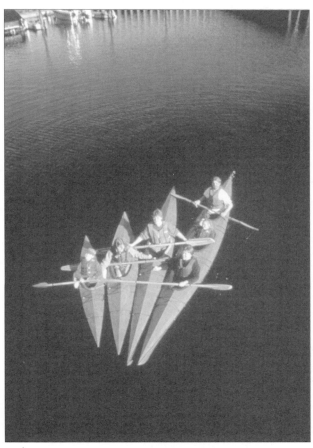

Wooden kayaks made from kits by Pygmy Boats come in all sizes. Shown are the Goldeneye 10', Goldeneye 13', Goldeneye standard, and the Osprey Triple. (Photo by John Lockwood, courtesy Pygmy Boats, Inc.)

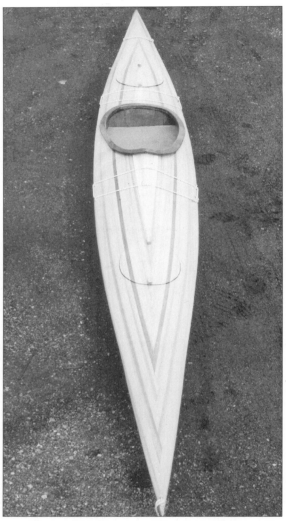

Elegant Tern (courtesy Woodstrip Watercraft)

The Kayak for You

Armed with the principles of design and materials, you must now decide which boat to buy from the bewildering number of models available. You don't have to decide alone. Most kayak dealers are experienced paddlers, and they can be very helpful in narrowing your search. Obviously, they have a product to sell, but those that stock several manufacturers' lines are usually less biased.

If you can find a local kayak club, you can meet and talk with people who have paddled a range of boats. If you're lucky, they may let you try their boats. Whatever you do, try to rent or test a demo boat before you buy it. A kayak's description on paper does not always match the way the boat paddles on the water. (See the back of this book for the appendix that lists paddling clubs in the United States and Canada.)

As you begin checking out kayaks, you can judge them against the design considerations spelled out earlier in this chapter. You'll check each boat's internal space—its volume—because this relates directly to its cargo capacity and to your comfort. You'll try the boats on for size, seeing if the cockpit suits your body.

You'll also assess the initial stability of the kayak—how it feels as it sits level in the water—and its secondary stability, which is the progressive stability of the boat as it is leaned onto its side. More stability as you lean means higher secondary stability. A kayak with good secondary stability is better able to handle waves, for instance.

If you're looking at a touring model, either a casual touring boat or a sea kayak for more serious touring, the issue of rudders

maneuverability, stability, hull efficiency, durability, and storage capacity. If a design attempts to maximize any one of these factors, other elements must be sacrificed to some extent. For example, kayaks designed just for speed can only be turned with the aid of a rudder, have no storage capacity, and can be kept upright only by an experienced paddler in calm conditions. Not exactly what you'd want in a whitewater kayak!

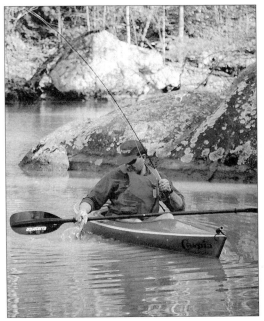

Touring with a Keowee (courtesy Perception)

and hatches becomes important. Does a rudder come standard with the boat? As an option? Is a skeg (a retractable fin on the bottom) available? Check out the size and watertightness of the storage hatches. (See the chapters on casual touring boats and sea kayaks for more details on rudders and hatches.)

Your overall plan in choosing a kayak might be summarized like this:

- Decide what kind of paddling you would like to do most of the time.
- Study as many different kayaks as possible in that class.
- Paddle the boat of your choice in as many conditions as possible.
- Assess the performance of the kayak in relation to its hull shape and weight.
- Talk to as many experienced paddlers as possible about their own boats.

Then you'll be ready to make the decision that's right for you.

Paddling Associations

The following are several associations dedicated to the promotion and improvement of paddle sports.

American Canoe Association
  7432 Alban Station Boulevard
  Suite B-226
  Springfield, VA 22150
  (703) 451–0141

American Whitewater Affiliation
  P.O. Box 636
  Margaret, NY 12455
  (914) 688–5569

Trade Association of Paddlesports
  12455 North Wauwatosa Road
  Mequon, WI 53097
  (414) 242–5228

Chapter 3
Choosing a Paddle

Selecting your paddle is a more complicated decision than you might think. This is because there is a wide range of designs, materials, and sizes from which to choose, and all these factors affect the performance and durability of the paddle.

Paddle Design

When choosing a paddle, you should examine the elements of paddle design—blade orientation, blade shape, blade size, and shaft shape.

Feathered or Unfeathered

The first question is whether you want the blades of the paddle to be feathered or unfeathered. These terms describe the orientation of the blades to one another.

- An unfeathered paddle has blades oriented in the same direction on each side.
- A feathered paddle has blades oriented perpendicular to one another. The idea behind the perpendicular orientation is that the blade out of the water will slice cleanly through the air.

If you choose feathered blades, you have to decide whether you want right-hand control (the most common) or left-hand control. If you choose right-hand control, for example, the grip of the right hand (the "control" hand) remains tight, though it flexes during the stroke. The grip of the left hand (called the "slip" hand) remains loose so the paddle can rotate in it. The opposite is true if you choose a left-hand control paddle. It's best to try both and see which is most comfortable.

Blade Shape

Blades can be flat or spooned. A flat blade is easier to handle because you can use either side for paddling. If the blade is shaped slightly like a spoon, it grabs the water better and flutters less when pulled through the water. When using a spooned blade, however, you have to be conscious of the blade because you cannot effectively use the back of the spooned paddle in making a stroke.

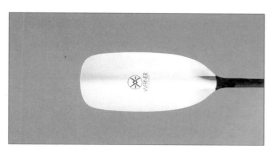

Ocoee, a kayak whitewater blade (courtesy Werner Paddles)

Blade Size

Is a bigger blade better? Large blades move more water and may give the impression of more power. But a smaller blade lets you move the blade faster and with less resistance on flat water or in wind.

Shaft

A blade shaft may be oval or round. Oval shafts feel more comfortable, and their ridges make it easier to orient the blade in the water.

Most kayak paddles have the standard, one-piece shaft in which the angle of the blade is fixed. Some paddles, however, are available in a take-apart version, which allows you to more easily transport and store the paddle as a spare (a good idea on remote trips); some take-apart models even allow you to change the angle of the blade.

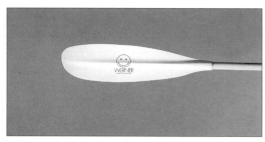

Point kids, proportionate-size fiberglass blade and shaft for smaller kayakers (courtesy Werner Paddles)

Paddle Length

There's no steadfast rule for selecting the length of a paddle, but it's a very important consideration nonetheless. The optimal length depends not only on your boat's dimensions and your body's dimensions but also on the type of kayaking you'll be doing. Whitewater kayaking typically uses shorter paddles than those for sea kayaking. Casual touring usually requires a paddle with a length somewhere in between.

The best advice is to talk to an experienced boater at the shop where you buy your kayak. If at all possible, try various paddle lengths (by renting or borrowing) before you buy a particular model.

Paddle Materials

Paddles, like boats, are made from a range of materials. Some verge on the downright exotic!

Wood

Wood paddles are the traditional choice among kayakers, and to many boaters no synthetic comes close to their beauty and flexibility. A good-quality wood paddle is expensive, however, and requires some maintenance.

Most wood paddles are made of laminated hardwoods, which are quite strong, even under pressure. Invariably, these paddles are fiberglassed or varnished to improve their durability. Many have sturdy tips of metal or fiberglass to prevent splitting under hard use.

Synthetics

Paddles can be made of materials such

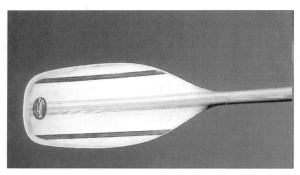

KMBS whitewater paddles (courtesy Sawyer Paddles & Oars)

as plastic (polypropylene), fiberglass, Kevlar, graphite, and carbon fiber. The lay-ups are as varied as the composites used in kayaks themselves.

It's possible to spend a great deal of money on high-tech materials, which offer light weight and good flexibility. Choose your paddle according to your need: Most sea kayakers and whitewater boaters find their needs more demanding than those who do casual touring.

Paddles for Sale

Following are descriptions of selected models from several kayak paddle manufacturers to give you an idea of what is avail-

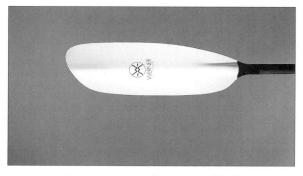

Camano, a popular touring blade (courtesy Werner Paddles)

able in whitewater and touring paddles. A comprehensive list of addresses and phone numbers for paddle manufacturers is given at the end of this chapter. Write to the manufacturers for their brochures, and talk with experienced paddlers to learn which models they use. With a bit of research, you'll inevitably choose the model that is right for your needs.

Ainsworth

Offers a number of paddles made of synthetics, including:
K106 Spec 2, Sea touring paddle with asymmetrical blade ($110).
K100 Spec 1, Whitewater slalom-type paddle ($90).
K104 Spec 5, Whitewater paddle with severe asymmetrical blade ($150).

Aqua-Bound

Offers a number of paddles made of synthetics, including:
Tripper, Touring paddle designed for long trips and for heavy loads ($75–$180, depending on materials).
Tsunami, full-size sea blade designed for power and acceleration ($105–$180, depending on materials).
Vortex, whitewater power paddle offering maximum acceleration and power ($105–$180, depending on materials).
Shred, whitewater paddle designed for serious playboating ($105–$180, depending on materials).

Grey Owl

Makes a line of wooden paddles, including:
Sirocco, very durable and dependable touring paddle ($125).
Tempest, extremely lightweight touring

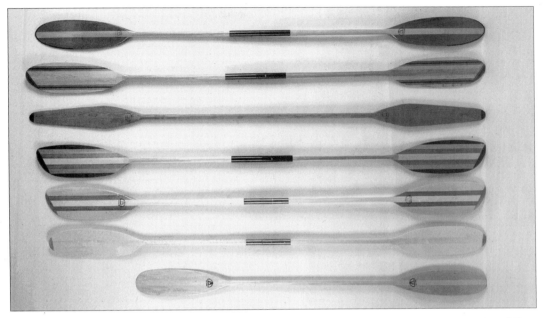

A selection from Grey Owl Paddles (courtesy Grey Owl Paddles)

paddle with pleasing flexibility ($140).

Spindrift, touring paddle ideal for long expeditions ($170).

Lightning

Offers a series of paddles made of synthetics, including:

Offshore, touring paddle with very narrow blades for reduced wind resistance ($205–$345, depending on materials).

Skimmer, asymmetrical touring paddle designed for power ($205–$345, depending on materials).

Standard Whitewater, whitewater paddle noted for its smooth curved blades and variety of fiberglass and graphite combinations ($110–$320, depending on materials).

Mitchell

Makes a number of wooden paddles, including:

Squirt, designed for the squirt boat specialist ($270).

Whitewater Play, for general whitewater playing ($215).

Nimbus

Offers a line of synthetic and wooden paddles, including:

Mystic, fiberglass touring paddle extolled for its durability and price ($105).

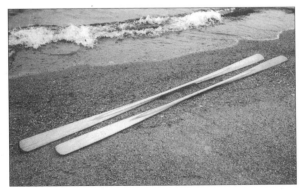

Handcarved Greenland paddles (courtesy Superior Kayaks)

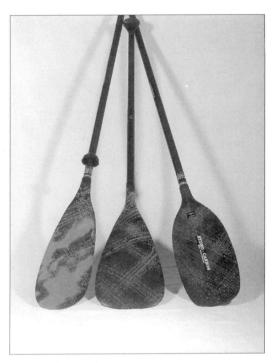

From left to right: K108 Spec 5, a touring paddle, C103 for canoeing, and the K104 Spec 5 whitewater Fibertech paddle, made of hydrocarbon (courtesy Ainsworth)

Seawater, wooden touring paddle with very broad blades ($175–$190).

Wavewalker, touring paddle available in fiberglass or graphite ($175–$190).

Perception, Inc.

Makes a number of synthetic and wooden paddles, including:

Gulfstream, narrow touring paddle available in fiberglass or graphite ($175–$260, depending on materials).

River Passage, whitewater paddle with nylon blades and composite-alloy shaft ($95–$105).

Shearwater, laminated wooden touring paddle noted for its lively feel ($150).

Paddle Manufacturers

Ainsworth
P.O. Box 207
Norwich, VT 05055
(802) 649–2952
Fax (802) 649–2254

Aqua-Bound Technology
#1-9520 192nd Street
Surrey, British Columbia V4N 3R8

In the U.S.:
1160 Yew Avenue
Blaine, WA 98230
(604) 882–2052
Fax (604) 882–9988

Backlund Paddles
26115 Clarksburg Road
Clarksburg, MD 20871
(301) 253–4947

Baldwin Boat Company
RR2, Box 268
Orrington, ME 04474-9611
(207) 825–4439

Baltic Paddles
330 McKinley Terrace
Centerport, NY 11721
(516) 673–4662
Fax (516) 673–8352

Bending Branches
812 Prospect Court
Osceola, WI 54020
(715) 755–3405
Fax (715) 755–3406

Betsie Bay Kayak
P.O. Box 1706
Frankfort, MI 49635
(616) 352–7774

Boreal Design
P.O. Box 37
St. Augustin, Quebec G3A 1V9
(418) 878–3099
Fax (418) 878–3459

Camp Paddle Company
2507 State Highway 7
Bainbridge, NY 13733
(607) 967–8755
E-mail: campadle@tri.town.net

Carlisle Paddles
P.O. Box 488
Grayling, MI 49738
(517) 348–9886
Fax (517) 348–8242

Caviness Woodworking Company
P.O. Box 710
Calhoun City, MS 38916
(601) 628–5195
Fax (601) 628–8580

Clinch River Paddle Company
2450 Jones Road
Lenoir City, TN 37771
(423) 986–9387

Cricket Paddles
17530 West Highway 50
Maysville
Salida, CO 81201
(719) 539–5010

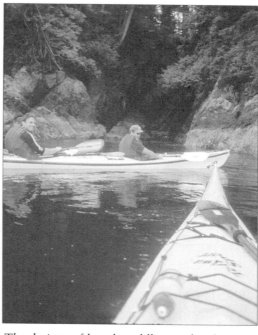

The designs of kayak paddles can be almost as specialized as kayaks themselves, and the final decision on which to use is largely a subjective one. (Courtesy Nimbus Paddles)

Current Designs
10124 McDonald Park Road
Sidney, British Columbia V8L 5X8

In the U.S.:
We-No-Nah Canoe Company
Box 247
Winona, MN 55987
(604) 655–1822
Fax (604) 655–1596
E-mail: info@cdkayak.com
Web: http://www.cdkayak.com

Dagger Canoe Company
P.O. Box 1500
Harriman, TN 37748
(423) 882–0404

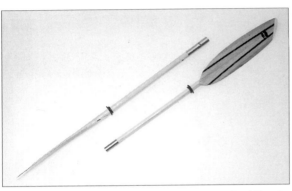

KSPS-FG paddle (courtesy Sawyer Paddles & Oars)

Epic Paddles
    6657 58th Avenue NE
    Seattle, WA 98115
    (206) 523–6306
    Fax (206) 523–6306

Far Horizon/Doctor D's
    P.O. Box 189

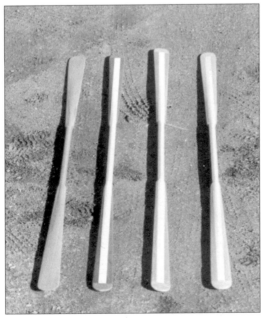

Greenland paddles (courtesy Woodstrip Watercraft Co.)

South Freeport, ME 04078
(207) 865–1244
(800) 295–0042

Glenwa
    P.O. Box 3134
    Gardena, CA 90247
    (310) 327–9216
    Fax (310) 327–8952
    E-mail: cobrakayaks@worldnet.att.net
    Web: http://www.cobrakayaks.com

Great Canadian Canoe Company
    64 Worcester Providence Turnpike
    Sutton, MA 01590
    (508) 865–0010
    Fax (508) 865–5220

Grey Owl Paddles
    62 Cowansview Road
    Cambridge, Ontario N1R 7N3
    (519) 622–0001
    Fax (519) 622–0723

Impex International/Formula Paddles
    1107 Station Road
    Bellport, NY 11713
    (516) 286–1988
    Fax (516) 286–1952

Janautica/Splashdance
    Highway 85 South
    Niceville, FL 32578
    (904) 678–1637
    Fax (904) 678–1637

L'eau Vive
    P.O. Box 18978
    Boulder, CO 80308
    (303) 417–1957
    Fax (303) 417–1446

Lee's Value Right
P.O. Box 19346
Minneapolis, MN 55419
(800) 758–1720
(612) 722–0057
Fax (612) 722–8040

Lendal Paddles/Great River Outfitters
4180 Elizabeth Lake Road
Waterford, MI 48328
(248) 683–4770
Fax (248) 683–0306

Lightning Paddles
22800 South Unger Road
Colton, OR 97017
(503) 824–2938
Fax (503) 824–6960

Malone of Maine
80 Second Street
South Portland, ME 04106
(207) 767–9776
Fax (207) 741–2477

Mitchell Paddles
RR 2, Box 922
Canaan, NH 03741
(603) 523–7004
Fax (603) 523–7363

Mohawk Paddles
963 North C.R. 427
Longwood, FL 32750
(407) 834–3233
Fax (407) 834–0292

Nimbus Paddles
4915 Chisholm Street
Delta, British Columbia
V4K 2K6

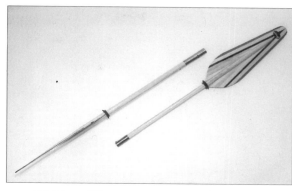

KSCA paddle (courtesy Sawyer Paddles & Oars)

(604) 526–2099
Fax (604) 522–1454

Norse Paddle Company
Route 1, Box 242
Spring Mills, PA 16875
(814) 422–8844
Fax (814) 422–8336

Northwest Design Works
(See Werner Paddles)

North Woods Canoe Company
Box 1419
Cochrane, Alberta, T0L 0W0
(403) 932–1948
Fax (403) 932–7123

Perception, Inc.
P.O. Box 8002
Easley, SC 29641
(800) 595–2925
Fax (864) 855–5995

Prijon/Wildwasser Sport USA
P.O. Box 4617
Boulder, CO 80306
(303) 444–2336
Fax (303) 444–2375

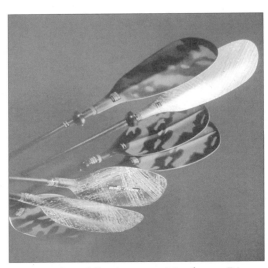

Ainsworth paddles (courtesy Northwest River Supplies)

Sawyer Paddles & Oars
299 Rogue River Parkway
Talent, OR 97540
(541) 535–3606
Fax (541) 535–3621

Seda Products
926 Coolidge Avenue
National City, CA 91950
(619) 336–2444

Sidewinder Whitewater
1692 Second Street
Richboro, PA 18954
(215) 598–3669

Silver Creek Paddles
677 Silvermine Road
Bryson City, NC 28713
(704) 488–9542
E-mail: silvrcrk@dnet.net

Superior Kayaks
108 Menasha
P.O. Box 355
Whitelaw, WI 54247
(414) 732–3784

Surfins
2227 Drake SW, #10A
Huntsville, AL 33805
(205) 882–2227
Fax (205) 551–9494

Swift/Eddyline Kayak Works
1344 Ashten Road
Burlington, WA 98233
(360) 757–2300
Fax (360) 757–2302

Tomic Golf & Ski Mfg.
23102 Mariposa Avenue
Torrance, CA 90502
(310) 534–2532
Fax (310) 534–2532

Twogood Kayaks Hawaii
345 Hahani Street
Kailua, HI 96734
(808) 262–5656
Fax (808) 261–3111
E-mail: twogood@alohoa.com

Venturesport
P.O. Box 610145
Miami, FL 33261
(561) 395–1376

Werner Paddles
P.O. Box 1139
Sultan, WA 98294
(800) 275–3311
Fax (360) 793–7343

Whispering Waters
    P.O. Box 497
    Mt. Shasta, CA 96067
    (916) 343–8681
    Fax: (916) 891–1433

Woodstrip Watercraft Com-
    pany
    1818 Swamp Pike
    Gilbertsville, PA 19525
    (610) 326–9282

ZuZu Paddle Company
    P.O. Box 957
    Flagstaff, AZ 86002
    (520) 774–6535
    Fax (520) 779–9466

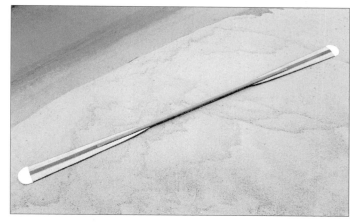

Greenlander style Graflite paddle (courtesy Betsie Bay Kayak)

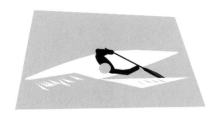

Chapter 4
Paddling Technique: The Basics

As a kayaker, you can make use of a wide range of strokes for propelling and turning your boat. The following is an introduction to the principal strokes. The introductions aren't meant to teach you how to perform the strokes; for this, check the list of books and tapes and the roster of paddling schools later in this chapter. These resources can help you attain the proper form and the most effective strokes.

Forward Stroke

This basic propulsion stroke is made powerful through a trunk-and-shoulder rotation. Accomplished kayakers will add some arm flexing, but the shoulder rotation is paramount. Keep this stroke precise and smooth.

Back Stroke

The back stroke is also a propulsion stroke, and it begins where the forward stroke ends. Because you don't insert the blade as far from your body as you do with a forward stroke, it's considerably less powerful.

Sweep Strokes

The sweep stroke—a forward or back stroke made in a wide, exaggerated arc away from the boat—is an effective turning stroke. There are two variations: the forward sweep and the reverse sweep.

Draw Stroke

The draw stroke is principally used for moving the kayak sideways. In executing the stroke, you reach out with the paddle and "draw" it straight toward you. The result is that the boat moves quickly toward the paddle.

Sculling Stroke

The sculling stroke is a holding stroke where the blade of the paddle is swept in a circular fashion to keep the boat in a stationary position. Since the blade never leaves the water, it's an efficient stroke.

Bracing Strokes

Bracing strokes are stabilizing strokes that keep the kayak from suddenly tipping over. The low brace—with the paddle held low—is actually a slap on the water that pushes you off the water to stabilize your position. The high brace—with the paddle held high—is more of a reaching motion that attempts to catch the water and thereby add stability.

Duffek Stroke

A more advanced stroke is the Duffek stroke (named after a famous paddler from Czechoslovakia named Milo Duffek). It is a very effective turning stroke that involves placing the paddle in the water by the bow of the boat. The paddler holds the paddle in that position, and the current literally swings the kayak around the paddle.

The Eskimo Roll

The Eskimo roll is a way of righting a kayak after it has capsized into an upside-

Instructional Videos

Paddling guru Kent Ford has produced a couple of instructional videos of interest to both sea kayakers and whitewater boaters: *Performance Sea Kayaking: The Basics and Beyond,* and *The Kayakers Edge* (whitewater boating).

They can be ordered from Four Corners River Sports, P.O. Box 379, Durango, CO 81302; (800) 426–7637.

down position. Mastery of the roll takes constant practice. While whitewater boaters are more likely to get regular practice than touring boaters, everyone could benefit from practicing the Eskimo roll—because you never know when you'll need it.

The maneuver is not difficult to master, but it does take work and, preferably, some guidance. Working with an experienced

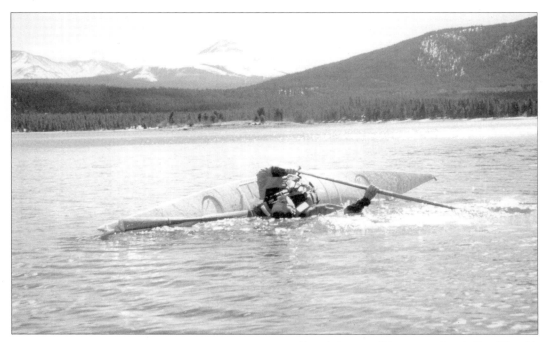

Practicing a roll (courtesy Betsie Bay Kayak)

kayaking instructor is without a doubt the best way to learn the skill. Some helpful books and videos are devoted to the subject.

As with most skills, there are a number of ways to do an Eskimo roll. Regardless of the roll you use, most are nothing more than a sweeping brace that happens to be performed upside down. The body is held close to the boat as you sweep the paddle out and then near the surface. Although it takes the entire body to accomplish the roll, it is really the action of the hips that causes the boat to flip over into the upright position.

Two excellent books to help you master the often elusive Eskimo roll are *Eskimo Rolling*, by Derek Hutchinson (London: A&C Black, 1999), and *The Bombproof Roll and Beyond*, by Paul Durky (Birmingham, Alabama: Menasha Ridge Press, 1997). A helpful video, *Grace Under Pressure*, is available from Great River Outfitters, 4180 Elizabeth Lake Road, Waterford, MI 48328; (248) 683–4770.

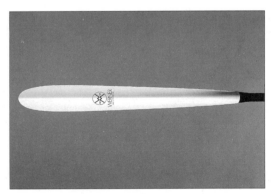

Arctic Wind, a combination of elements from old and new Aleut and West Greenland paddles, perfect for Eskimo paddling styles (courtesy Werner Paddles)

Paddling Strokes

"A kayak is a water vehicle powered by a person wielding a paddle. Every movement of the craft, in whatever direction, is due to the paddle being held in a certain position and moved in a certain manner. We call these maneuvers the *basic strokes*. The term can be misleading, because it invites the reader to suppose that there are other strokes which are more advanced; whereas, in fact, when we refer to *advanced strokes* we are really only talking about the basic strokes performed in a more professional manner, in a smooth sequence, or in a more demanding or 'advanced' situation."

—Derek C. Hutchinson
The Complete Book of Sea Kayaking

Paddling Schools

One of the best ways to learn good paddling technique is with the help of a qualified instructor.

Ace Paddling Center
P.O. Box 1168
Oak Hill, WV 25901
(800) 787–3982

Adventure Quest
P.O. Box 184
Woodstock, VT 05091
(802) 484–3939

Boulder Outdoor Center
2510 North 47th Street
Boulder, CO 80301
(800) 364–9376
(303) 444–8420

Paddle Humor

Teaching kayak technique with cartoons? Paddle humorist (and experienced kayaker) William Nealy provides solid tips on running whitewater in his book *Kayak: The Animated Manual of Intermediate and Advanced Whitewater Technique* (Birmingham, Alabama: Menasha Ridge Press, 1997). This is bizarre off-the-wall humor, but good fun.

If you like this one, try Nealy's other kayaking books: *Kayaks to Hell* and *Whitewater Tales of Terror* (both also from Menasha Ridge Press).

California Canoe and Kayak School
 11257 South Bridge Street
 Rancho Cordova, CA 95670
 (800) 366–9804

Current Adventures Kayak School
 1800 Twitchell Road
 Placerville, CA 95667
 (916) 642–9755

Endless River Adventures
 P.O. Box 246
 Bryson City, NC 28713
 (704) 488–6199

George Gronseth's Kayak Academy
 2512 NE 95th Street
 Seattle, WA 98115
 (206) 527–1825

H2Outfitters
 P.O. Box 72
 Orr's Island, ME 04066
 (800) 205–2925

Jackson Hole Kayak School
 P.O. Box 9201
 Jackson Hole, WY 83001
 (800) 733–2471

Kayak & Canoe Institute
 University of Minnesota at Duluth
 Outdoor Center
 121 SpHC, 10 University Drive
 Duluth, MN 55812
 (218) 726–6533

Kayak Centre
 9 Phillips Street
 Wickford, RI 02852
 (401) 295–4400

Maine Island Kayak Company
 70 Luther Street
 Peaks Island, ME 04108
 (800) 796–2373
 (207) 766–2373

Nantahala Outdoor Center

It has been called "the Harvard of paddling schools" by *Esquire* magazine, and almost everyone in the paddling world knows of the NOC near Wesser, North Carolina, and Great Smoky Mountains National Park.

Founded in the early 1970s in an old motel and gas station on the banks of the Nantahala River, NOC is now a bustling community that offers kayaking instruction (whitewater and touring) and an interesting range of guided trips, both at home and abroad. (Nantahala Outdoor Center, 13077 Highway 19 West, Bryson City, NC 28713; 704–488–6737).

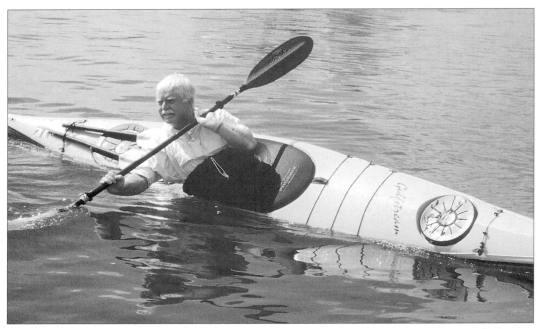

Derek Hutchinson demonstrates his technique (courtesy Current Designs/We-no-nah Canoe)

Mandawaska Kanu Centre
  Box 635
  Barry's Bay, Ontario K0J 1B0
  (613) 594–5268
  (613) 756–3620

Nantahala Outdoor Center
  13077 Highway 19 West
  Bryson City, NC 28713
  (704) 488–6737

North American River Runners
  P.O. Box 81
  Hico, WV 25854
  (800) 950–2585

Otter Bar Kayak School
  Box 210
  Forks of Salmon, CA 96031
  (916) 462–4772

River Run Paddling Centre
  P.O. Box 179
  Beachburg, Ontario K0J 1C0
  (613) 646–2501

Riversport School of Paddling
  P.O. Box 95
  213 Yough Street
  Confluence, PA 15424
  (814) 395–5744

Sierra South Mountain Sports
  P.O. Box Y
  Kernville, CA 93239
  (619) 376–3745

Snake River Kayak and Canoe School
  P.O. Box 3482
  Jackson, WY 83001
  (800) 529–2501

Sundance Kayak School
14894 Galice Road
Merlin, OR 97532
(541) 479–8508

Whitewater Challengers Outdoor
Adventure Center
P.O. Box 8
White Haven, PA 18661
(717) 443–9532

W.I.L.D./W.A.T.E.R.S. Outdoor Center
Route 28, The Glen
Warrensburg, NY 12885
(800) 867–2335

Zoar Outdoor
P.O. Box 245
Charlemont, MA 01339
(800) 532–7483

Good Reads: Kayaking Technique

The following are some general introductory books on kayak technique. More books are listed within the chapters that cover the various types of kayaking.

The Kayaking Book (second edition), by Eric Evans and Jay Evans (New York: Plume/New American Library/Penguin Books, 1993): a must-read for those interested in whitewater boating, authored by two of the best instructors in the sport.

Kayaking Made Easy, by Dennis Stuhaug (The Globe Pequot Press, 1998): clearly written instructions on touring technique.

The Complete Book of Sea Kayaking, by Derek C. Hutchinson (The Globe Pequot Press, 1995): A well-illustrated guide.

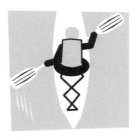

Chapter 5
Casual Touring Boats

Kayaks designed for casual touring are asked to do just about everything—maintain good stability, perform well at tracking, carry big loads when needed, endure heavy waves at times, and yet remain relatively easy and fast to paddle. Many casual touring boats are made for a single paddler, but two-person kayaks (called a K-2) are also produced in which one paddler sits directly behind the other. Some K-2 models have one large open cockpit; in others, separate cockpits are provided.

A casual recreation or touring kayak is defined by function more than form. Most paddlers prefer a boat that paddles easily, will handle rough water when it has to, and is suited to their style of paddling and cargo needs.

Design Considerations

Most people looking at casual touring kayaks want a boat that is relatively stable under most conditions. Naturally, they want a kayak that will move ahead efficiently and

track in a straight line. Constant corrections to keep the boat heading on course waste energy that could be used to keep the boat moving ahead. So designers lay out relatively long hulls for touring kayaks because they are faster and track better. A touring kayak will resist turning more than a shorter hull of similar width. If you paddle a short kayak and a longer touring kayak back-to-back, you will notice that the bow of the shorter boat moves off course more readily with each stroke than the longer one does.

The keel (the bottom profile from bow to stern) of most touring boats is either a straight line or upturned somewhat. The middle serves as a pivot point, allowing the boat to turn. It's a tradeoff: boats that track well are harder to turn, whereas boats that turn easily are harder to paddle in a straight line.

For most purposes, boats designed for casual recreational touring will have hull shapes and dimensions that hover around a norm. You should avoid extremes of design or dimension, unless you have a specialized need that demands a significant departure from the norm.

Consider the cross-sectional view of the bottom, for example. A kayak with a nearly flat bottom will be very stable when it is floating level. However, if the boat is forced up on edge, there will come a point at which it will abruptly flip over. A more rounded hull is often associated with an unstable boat. Yet if you rock that hull over on its side, it becomes more stable and buoyant, and it gives you plenty of advance warning before going completely over. Most touring boats keep to the mid-range of shapes, commonly having a shallow-V bottom or a shallow arch bottom (slightly rounded), rather than one that is flat or heavily rounded.

Special Features

With a boat designed for overnight touring, you'll need to consider a few special features. (Also see Chapter 6, on sea kayaks, for discussion of other features that could be helpful on a casual touring boat, depending on your intended use, including compass and light, retractable skeg, and deck-fitted bilge pump.)

Hatches and Bulkheads

The greatest innovation in touring kayak design in recent years has been the introduction of watertight hatches and bulkheads. Equipment can be kept dry at all times, and the boat is virtually unsinkable. Any hatch that allows entry into the interior of a kayak should be watertight, and designed so that it cannot be knocked off.

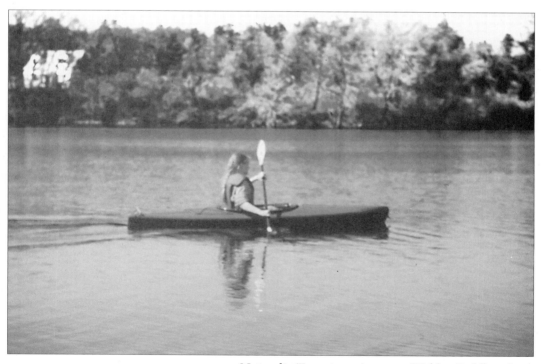

Naturalist/Experience (courtesy Walden Paddlers, Inc.)

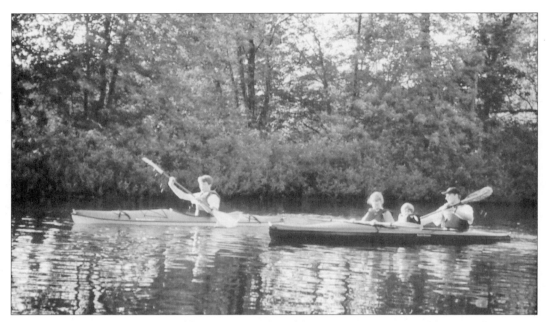

Walden Vision and Walden Spirit (courtesy Walden Paddlers, Inc.)

There is nothing wrong with a large hatch opening, as long as it remains watertight.

Rudder

Paddlers often debate whether kayaks should have rudders, and often the decision depends upon the kayak design. Some kayaks are specifically designed not to need a rudder.

Rudders can undoubtedly be an advantage for some designs. Turning is clearly easier with the aid of a rudder. The difficulty of tracking in a tandem kayak is probably best corrected by using a rudder. This does away with the necessity of leaning the boat over onto one side, which is much more difficult with two paddlers than one.

Many solo paddlers who depend on rudders at the beginning of their careers tend to use them less as their skill level increases. For example, paddlers usually learn quickly that most touring kayaks can be turned

easily by taking advantage of the waves: The boat is spun around by the paddle as the hull pirouettes on top of a wave.

The purists dislike rudders because they can break, get fouled up in nets or lines, and inhibit landings and launchings.

Tandem Kayaks

Kayaks that carry two paddlers—called tandems, or doubles—offer a number of advantages. Two paddlers of equal strength and skill can go faster and farther and travel more efficiently if they are paddling one tandem kayak rather than a pair of solos. A tandem, because it is almost always wider and longer, is more stable than a single of equal design. And a tandem allows paddlers of differing strengths and skills to travel more easily together, since the weaker paddler isn't forced to catch up in his or her own boat.

A child can come along in the bow cockpit of a tandem. A few designs even have a third cockpit, allowing the child to sit in the middle, with adults on either end. A tandem also gives you the option of transporting a tired or injured solo paddler by having one of the tandem kayakers trade places with the paddler in the one-person boat. But the best reason of all for a tandem is the camaraderie that can develop between the two boaters, who are able to carry on a conversation while wielding the paddles.

Tandem boats—especially ones with a center cockpit—can obviously carry more gear than can a single kayak. Even a double-burner Coleman stove will fit inside the bigger models. This carrying capacity is a big advantage, but don't be misled into thinking a double can carry twice as much as a single. Two solo boats can easily and efficiently carry more weight than one double kayak.

Tandem boats, because they are larger and are controlled by two minds instead of just one, are less maneuverable than a solo boat. But in big waves, a tandem is tremendously more stable. Being larger, a tandem

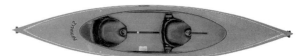

Perception's Keowee 2

can also fill up with more water, making it impossible to move. For that reason, you'll need to make sure that it has proper flotation.

Finding the Right Boat

Choosing the best casual touring boat for your purposes involves the same general process that was outlined earlier for selecting any kayak. As you look at touring models:

- Decide what kind of paddling you will do most of the time. Do you expect to stay in calm water? Will you be trying coastal cruising?
- Study as many different kayaks as you can that seem to meet your needs.
- Paddle the boat of your choice under a variety of conditions.
- Assess performance in relation to the

Superior Images

Several beautiful books are devoted to kayaking on Michigan's Lake Superior, a popular touring destination.

The Lake Superior Images, by Craig Blacklock (Moose Lake, Minnesota: Blacklock Nature Photography, 1993)

Superior: Journeys on an Inland Sea, by Gary and Joannie McGuffin (Minocqua, Wisconsin: Northword Press, 1995)

Lake Superior's North Shore & Isle Royale, by Kate Crowley (Stillwater, Minnesota: Voyageur Press, 1989)

Superior: The Haunted Shore, by Bruce Littlejohn and Wayland Drew (New York: Firefly Books, 1995)

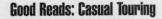

Good Reads: Casual Touring

As you can see by the titles of some of the books and videos listed in this chapter, casual touring boats are also used for sea kayaking (which is the subject of the next chapter). The main difference is one of degree. The casual touring boats are more often used on quiet rivers, sheltered waters, and moderate coastal areas. The sea kayaks used for more serious touring tend to be somewhat longer, more durable craft used on extended travels, rougher waters, or the open sea.

There are a number of excellent books on recreational touring. Here's a list, beginning with the most basic and progressing to the more advanced.

Sea Kayaking Basics, by David Harrison (New York: Hearst Marine Books, 1993)
The Essential Sea Kayaker: A Complete Course for the Open Water Paddler, by David Seidman (Camden, Maine: Ragged Mountain Press, 1992)
Kayaking Made Easy, by Dennis Stuhaug (The Globe Pequot Press, 1998)
The Coastal Kayaker's Manual (third edition), by Randel Washburne (The Globe Pequot Press, 1998)

---

kayak's hull shape and weight.

• Talk to experienced paddlers about their own boats.

As you look at boats, remember that all designs are a compromise of sorts, and that ultimately the decision is a subjective one. If you're planning, for example, to paddle across placid lakes on afternoon outings, you may be more concerned with stability than cargo capacity. On the other hand, if you're planning extended trips down wilderness rivers, you'll need a boat that provides generous space for gear. And of course there are many other models for the wide range of trips that recreational kayakers take. In any event, it's always a good idea to try before you buy.

Wind and Waves

Once you have the paddling strokes down, the biggest obstacles to safe, comfortable touring are wind and waves. They can be just as much a hazard on a lake as rocks and rapids are on a river.

Headwinds

Kayakers need to study the techniques for paddling into headwinds in order to keep the boat from capsizing. Looking at a map or at the crossing itself for protection from the wind is an important precaution, as is studying the possibilities for escape if the wind should pick up to dangerous levels.

To hold a kayak on course while heading into the wind, it's best to paddle with quick and effective paddle strokes. As waves increase in size and force, the best precaution is to turn the bow straight into the wind to avoid being pushed into a more vulnerable sideways position. When large whitecaps start to appear on the waves, the situation is more hazardous, and it's time to seek shelter.

Crosswinds

Paddling in crosswinds requires yet an-

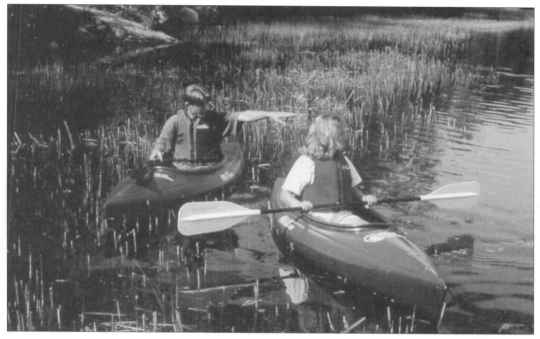

Otter (courtesy Old Town Canoe)

other set of tactics. Even in a light cross-wind, you may be blown sideways and, as a result, arrive far from your intended destination. Increasing crosswinds bring with them the danger of being rolled over.

To avoid these problems, you need to angle into the waves, in a movement known as quartering the waves. In really large waves, the bow must be turned directly into the waves to avoid capsizing.

Tailwinds

Many paddlers think that tailwinds don't present a problem because the wind is at their backs. This may be the case in light winds, but as the waves increase, tailwinds can become very challenging.

In strong tailwinds, the wave pushes the stern up and the fast-moving kayak buries its bow into the wave ahead. As the wave

passes underneath the kayak, it tends to push the boat to one side, making a capsize more likely. A strong rudder or draw stroke is necessary to keep the kayak on course.

Lake Crossings

On large, windy lakes, it's important for

Instructional Videos

Paddling technique for casual touring is well demonstrated by expert Kent Ford in the video *Performance Sea Kayaking: The Basics and Beyond.* Another excellent how-to video is *Sea Kayaking* (Trailside Series).

Both can be ordered from Four Corners River Sports, P.O. Box 379, Durango, CO 81302; (800) 426–7637.

Arctic Voyage

Among the Inuit people, Victoria Jason became known as the *kabloona*, the Inuktikuk word for stranger. In the summer of 1991, Jason, a novice kayaker, began an Arctic voyage that would eventually entail 4,500 miles and consume four summers.

Despite a number of lingering medical problems, Jason set out from Churchill, Manitoba, and paddled the first half of the journey to Gjoa Haven on King William Island. She completed the circle by then starting at Fort Providence on Great Slave Lake and heading up the Mackenzie River to its mouth, and then paddling along the coast through the Beaufort Sea back to Gjoa Haven. The tale is contained in her book *Kabloona in the Yellow Kayak* (Winnipeg: Turnstone Press, 1995).

safety for kayakers to stay together. The best plan is to designate an experienced paddler to stay in front of the group. This lead boater can set the pace, determine the route, and call for rest stops. It's also a good idea to have an experienced kayaker in a "sweep" boat bringing up the rear, ready to help anyone having trouble. If there are no rest stops, it's advisable to wait for slower paddlers by pointing your kayak into the wind and paddling just hard enough to hold your position.

Safety Gear for Casual Touring

A number of devices make life on the water a little safer as you travel in a casual touring boat. (See Chapter 15 for a fuller discussion of safety equipment).

Personal flotation device. The PFD is your most indispensable piece of safety equipment.

Bilge pump. Make sure it's securely fastened to the boat.

Compass. A good marine compass is indispensable, and many touring kayaks allow for mounting of a compass on the deck.

Flashing beacons, flares, and smoke devices. If you get into trouble, you need some sort of device to alert others.

Whistle. For person-to-person alerts.

First-aid kit. Imperative, especially for longer and more remote trips.

Gloves. To prevent the blisters that can ruin a trip.

The Builders

Among the manufacturers of casual touring boats (recreational kayaks) are Old Town and Wilderness Systems, and some of their boats are discussed here. You'll find statistical details on casual touring boats made by these and other manufacturers in the fact grids that follow this section.

The Indispensable Compass

"Every kayaker should carry a compass on anything beyond a 'backyard' trip. Though I have used my compass only a handful of times in a dozen years of paddling, I would have had significant problems without it; I have cut short more than one trip because I left my compass at home. I now carry a compass whenever I paddle."

—Randel Washburne
The Coastal Kayaker's Manual

Old Town

Old Town Canoe Company, based in Old Town, Maine, has been building boats since 1898. The company's traditional business was in canoes, of course, but its line of kayaks, especially casual recreation boats, is expanding rapidly. All of its casual touring boats are made of polyethylene.

The flagship of Old Town's recreational touring boats is the Loon 138, which is 13 feet, 8 inches long and made of Polylink 3 polyethylene. A large open cockpit allows a child or pet to come along for the ride. This is a stable yet efficient solo kayak with a folding, high-back bucket seat. The Loon 138 uses Old Town's roto-molded process to produce a tough three-layered polyethylene hull, which contributes to a stiffer bottom and deck while reducing weight and omitting the need for a keel. The foam core provides built-in flotation, and also acts as insulation against cold and noise. An optional rudder is available. Weight is 54 pounds. Price: about $500.

The Loon 138T is the tandem version of the Loon 138. This model offers the additional space of a tandem model, but with the better maneuverability and handling of a shorter design (it's the same length as the Loon 138). The 138T is a good boat for an adult and child, and it's a manageable size for people with small cars or limited storage space. Weighing 59 pounds, the boat comes with two high-back folding seats with adjustable backstraps, stern deck rigging, and two kayak paddle holders. An optional rudder is available. Price: about $600.

The Loon 160T, a 16-foot tandem boat weighing 74 pounds, comes in a generous size that allows the family to get out on the water in a stable yet efficient design. Adding to the comfort is the large nonconfining cockpit and folding high-seat back. This tandem switches to a solo by sliding the bow seat. The cockpit of the 160T can accommodate extra gear, a small third person, or a pet. An optional rudder is available. Price: about $650.

The Loon 120 (12 feet long and 49 pounds) is a smaller, easier-to-handle version of the Loon 138. Its width of 28 inches provides good stability. The Loon 120 is a reasonable candidate for boaters looking for a kayak that is easy to carry and load on a vehicle. Price: $450.

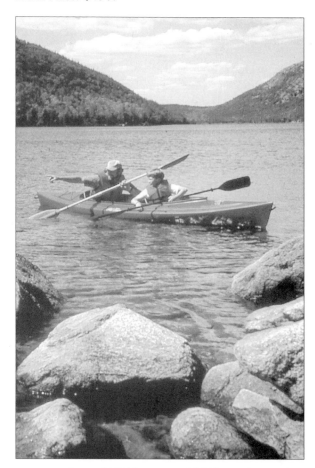

Loon 138T (courtesy Old Town Canoe Co.)

Kayaks for Kids

Children are beginning to paddle at amazingly early ages, and many manufacturers, such as Perception, Inc., offer boats designed for children. One company, Englehart Products Inc. (EPI), of Newbury, Ohio, offers an extensive line of boats just for children. See the manufacturers' list at the end of this chapter for the addresses of Perception and Englehart.

Boaters have a good general recreation kayak in the basic model in Old Town's Otter Series. It is 9 feet, 6 inches long and weighs 39 pounds—comfortable, stable, and easy to paddle. The high-back seat is comfortable, and a large cockpit allows for easy entry and exit. Because it is small and lightweight, the Otter is easy to carry or to transport on a cartop. Price: $300.

Wilderness Systems

Wilderness Systems, based in Archdale, North Carolina, has been producing touring kayaks since 1986. It now offers one of the most extensive lines in the business. Its casual recreation boats are made of polyethylene and are quite stable, designed well for people who like to fish, bird-watch, or simply cruise.

The Rascal is 9 feet, 8 inches long and weighs 40 pounds. Designed by veteran kayaker Joe Walton, the Rascal's 30-inch width works well for younger paddlers or for older ones who prefer a solid, stable feel

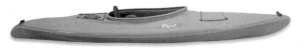

Wilderness System's Rascal

on the water. The Rascal is light, easily portable, and capable of going where bigger boats can't: ponds, mangrove swamps, tidal creeks—and out of the way in the garage. Simple deck bungies make it easy to store gear on top of the kayak. Price: about $450.

The Pungo, also designed by Walton, looks like an extended Rascal. It weighs 50 pounds and is just over 12 feet long, giving more legroom and a bigger cockpit. An up-

Wilderness System's Pamlico Lite

swept bow helps with wave-piercing capabilities and speed, while a recurved stern keeps Pungo on track. Deck bungies are standard. Price: about $550.

The Pamlico and Pamlico Lite are tandem models noted for comfort while retaining swiftness and maneuverability. The roomy cockpit in this design by John Shep-

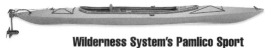

Wilderness System's Pamlico Sport

pard aids entry and exit. A big advantage of the Pamlico is its ability to carry a week's worth of gear. Depending on size and on whether you choose polyethylene, fiberglass, or Kevlar, the price varies: $700–$1900.

The 16-foot, 70-pound Pamlico Excel is known as a sport utility vehicle for the water. Ample storage fore and aft keeps gear out of the weather. An optional foot-controlled rudder is available. This is both a single and a tandem—and there's even room

Guidebooks: Kayak Touring

Following are some of the more noteworthy guidebooks for coastal touring by kayak. Depending on the demands of the trip, these guidebooks are applicable to either casual touring boats or sea kayaks.

Guide to Sea Kayaking in Central and Northern California: The Best Trips from Morro Bay to the Lost Coast, by Roger Schumann (Old Saybrook, Conn.: The Globe Pequot Press, 1999)

Guide to Sea Kayaking in Southern Florida: The Best Trips from Sarasota to Key West, by Nigel Foster (Old Saybrook, Conn.: The Globe Pequot Press, 1999)

Kayaking Puget Sound: The San Juans and Gulf Islands, by Randel Washburne (Seattle: The Mountaineers, 1990)

Sea Kayaking Canada's West Coast, by John Ince and Heidi Kottner (Seattle: The Mountaineers, 1992)

Sea Kayaking in Baja, by Andromeda Romano-Lax (Berkeley: Wilderness Press, 1993)

Sea Kayaking in Florida, by David Gluckman (Sarasota: Pineapple Press, 1995)

Sea Kayaking the Carolinas, by James Bannon and Morrison Giffen (Out There Publishers, 1997)

Sea Kayaking in the Florida Keys, by Bruce Wachob (Sarasota: Pineapple Press, 1997)

Sea Kayaking the Mid-Atlantic Coast, by Tamsin Venn (Boston: Appalachian Mountain Club Books, 1994)

Sea Kayaking the New England Coast, by Tamsin Venn (Boston: Appalachian Mountain Club Books, 1991)

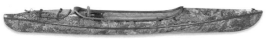

Wilderness System's Chesapeake

for three with the standard child seat. Price: about $750.

The Chesapeake, also designed by Sheppard, is 12 feet, 4 inches long and weighs 36 pounds. It is known for quickness and sta-bility, and works well for boaters who carry a lot of gear. It can be ordered in a camouflage color, the official pattern of Ducks Unlimited, which helps you maintain a low profile on the marshes. Or you can choose from a selection of brilliant gel-coat finishes. Price: fiberglass ($1250); Kevlar ($1750).

Casual Touring Boats

The following grids present details on the lineup of casual touring boats offered by selected manufacturers. See the end of this chapter for the addresses and phone numbers of these and other manufacturers. For information on paddles, see Chapter 3. For information on spray skirts, life jackets, and other accessories, see Chapter 14.

Manufacturer/model	Length (feet)	Width (inches)	Weight (pounds)	Material
Baldwin (1966)				
Family K-2 (tandem)	14'	38	60	fiberglass
Sailing K-2 (tandem)	14'	38	72	fiberglass
Dagger (1988)				
Bayou	10'8"	28	42	polyethylene
Bayou 2 (Tandem)	14'	30	65	polyethylene
Editso	14'6"	24½	49	polyethylene
Seeker	16'	23½	52	polyethylene
Vesper	13'10"	24	46	polyethylene
Englehart (1988)				
Episea (designed for women)	14'2"	20½	38	polyethylene
Epitour	14'	25	38	polyethylene
Futura (1987)				
Spear	16'	19	35	polyethylene
Great Canadian (1972)				
Rainbow	13'	24	46	polyethylene
River Runner R5	13'	24	35	polyethylene
Hobie Cat (1968)				
Odyssey	14'	33	80	polyethylene
Pursuit	12'	28	47	polyethylene
Hop On Top (1995)				
12' HopOnTop	12'	27	32	fiberglass
Hydra (1992)				
Minnow	8'9"	29	41	polyethylene
Janautica/Splashdance (1983)				
Alaska-PO	15'	24	50	polyethylene
JK Inc (1973)				
Canyak AH1	10'6"	27	45	fiberglass (chopped)
Canyak AL1	10'6"	27	40	fiberglass (chopped)
Canyak AL3	10'6"	27	40	fiberglass (chopped)
Canyak E1	13'	31	60	fiberglass (chopped)
Canyak E3	13'	31	55	fiberglass (chopped)
Kiwi (1988)				
Kapapa	8'8"	27	33	polyethylene
Lobo	9'2"	29	37	polyethylene
Lobo Gato	9'2"	29	37	polyethylene
Mark 4	13'6"	29	61	polyethylene
Mark Twain	13'6"	29	61	polyethylene
Mainstream (1996)				
Jazz	9'	30	35	polyethylene
Tango	12'	34	52	polyethylene
Necky (1983)				
Gannet II	14'9"	30	78	polyethylene
Santa Cruz	12'5"	29	47	polyethylene

Keel	Bottom	Sides	Price (dollars)
straight ends	shallow V	straight	950
straight ends	shallow V	straight	1600
straight with rise at ends	shallow V	flared	500
straight with rise at ends	shallow V	flared	700
moderate rocker	shallow arch	flared	750
moderate rocker	shallow arch	flared	800
moderate rocker	shallow arch	flared	700
straight with rise at ends	shallow arch	flared	600
straight with rise at ends	shallow V	flared	600
extreme rocker	shallow arch	flared	1150
straight with rise at ends	flat	straight	300-400*
moderate rocker	shallow arch	flared	600
moderate rocker	rounded V	straight	750
moderate rocker	rounded V	straight	600
moderate rocker	shallow arch	straight	1,000
straight with rise at ends	shallow V	straight	400
straight with rise at ends	rounded V	tumblehome	700
straight	rounded V	straight	450
straight	rounded V	straight	450
straight with rise at ends	rounded V	straight	450
extreme rocker	flat	straight	600
extreme rocker	flat	straight	600
straight with rise at ends	shallow arch	straight	450
straight with rise at ends	shallow V	straight	450
straight with rise at ends	shallow V	straight	1050
straight with rise at ends	shallow V	straight	1350
straight with rise at ends	shallow V	straight	650
moderate rocker	shallow arch	straight	350
moderate rocker	shallow arch	straight	500
moderate rocker	shallow arch	flared	700-1000*
moderate rocker	shallow arch	flared	550-800*

Manufacturer/model	Length (feet)	Width (inches)	Weight (pounds)	Material
Old Town (1898)				
Loon Series (including tandem)	12', 13'8", 16'	28¾-29½	49-74*	polyethylene
Otter Series	9'6"	28½	39-42*	polyethylene
Perception (1975)				
Aquaterra Caspia	10'4"	29	40	polyethylene
Aquaterra Jocassee	16'6"	32½	85	polyethylene
Aquaterra Keowee Series				
(including tandem)	9'2", 12'10"	29, 32½	42-66*	polyethylene
Swifty 3.1	9'5"	29	37	polyethylene
Phoenix Poke Boats (1973)				
Poke Boat	12'	32	22-28*	proprietary lay-up or Kevlar
Poke Boat Maxi Series	11'10", 18'8"	37	27-32*	proprietary lay-up or Kevlar
Poke Boat Micro	7'11"	35	14-17*	proprietary lay-up or Kevlar
Prijon (1985)				
Taifun Tour	12'9"	24	50	polyethylene
Seda (1969)				
Vagabond	14'	25	29-43	fiberglass or Kevlar
Swift (1994)				
Tasman Sea	13'6"	25	32	proprietary lay-up
The Upstream Edge (1984)				
Q-Star	10'	30	25	fiberglass
Tsunami (1986)				
X-2 Starship (tandem)	19'10"	29	90	Kevlar
Valhalla (1983)				
Valhalla	19'	19¾	35	fiberglass
Viking International	19'	19¼	32	fiberglass
Vermont Canoe Products (1989)				
Expedition	14'	24	37	fiberglass
Expedition II	14'	24	40	fiberglass
Salmon	13'4"	23½	53	fiberglass
Walden (1992)				
Experience	10'	27	35	polyethylene
Naturalist	12'	27	34	polyethylene
Spirit (tandem)	14'	30	63	polyethylene
Wilderness Systems (1986)				
Chesapeake	12'4"	32	31-36*	fiberglass or Kevlar
Manteo	13'	27	50	polyethylene
Pamlico Series	14'5", 15'1",	29½, 30½,		fiberglass, Kevlar,
(including tandem)	16'	32	44-85*	or polyethylene
Pungo	12'1"	29	50	polyethylene
Rascal	9'8"	30	40	polyethylene

(Year in parentheses is year the company began making boats)
* Depending on model, material, or options

Keel	Bottom	Sides	Price (dollars)
straight with rise at ends	shallow V or round V	tumblehome or flared	450-650*
straight with rise at ends	shallow V	tumblehome	300-400*
straight with rise at ends	flat	flared	500
straight with rise at ends	shallow arch	flared	750
straight with rise at ends	shallow V	straight	450-650*
straight with rise at ends	flat	flared	350
straight	flat	flared	950-1300*
straight	flat	flared	1050-2050*
straight	flat	flared	500-800*
moderate rocker	shallow arch	tumblehome	750
straight with rise at ends	shallow arch	flared	800-1100*
moderate rocker	rounded V	flared	1600
straight ends	shallow V	straight	600
moderate rocker	shallow V	flared	3500
extreme rocker	shallow V	straight	1100
moderate rocker	shallow V	straight	2000
moderate rocker	shallow arch	tumblehome	700
moderate rocker	shallow arch	tumblehome	850
moderate rocker	shallow arch	straight	600
straight with rise at ends	shallow arch	flared	500
straight with rise at ends	shallow arch	flared	450
straight with rise at ends	shallow arch	flared	700
straight	flat	flared	1250-1750*
moderate rocker	shallow V	flared	650
moderate rocker	shallow V	flared	700-1900*
moderate rocker	shallow V	flared	550
moderate rocker	shallow V	flared	450

Manufacturers of Casual Touring Boats

Baldwin Boat Company
RR 2, Box 268
Orrington, ME 04474
(207) 825–4439

Chesapeake Light Craft
1805 George Avenue
Annapolis, MD 21401
(410) 267–0137
Fax (301) 858–6335

Dagger Canoe Company
P.O. Box 1500
Harriman, TN 37748
(423) 882–0404
Fax (423) 882–8153

Englehart Products Inc. (EPI)
P.O. Box 377
Newbury, OH 44065
(216) 564–5565
Fax (216) 564–5515

Futura Surf Skis
730 West 19th Street
National City, CA 91950
(619) 474–8382
Fax (619) 474–5167

Great Canadian Canoe Company
64 Worcester Providence Turnpike
Sutton, MA 01590

(508) 865–0010
Fax (508) 865–5220

Hobie Cat Company (Outback Division)
4925 Oceanside Boulevard
Oceanside, CA 92056
(760) 758–9100 ext. 400
Fax (760) 758–1841

Hop On Top Kayaks
P.O. Box 139
Jamestown, RI 02835
(401) 423–1815
Fax (401) 423–1815

Hydra Kayaks
5061 South National Drive
Knoxville, TN 37914
(800) 537–8888
Fax (305) 836–1296

Janautica/Splashdance
Highway 85 South
Niceville, FL 32578
(850) 678–1637
Fax (850) 678–1637
Web: http://www.splashdance.com

JK Inc.
207 1/2 Franklin Street North
Ackley, IA 50601-1254
(515) 847–2151
Fax (515) 847–2218

Kiwi Kayak Company
2454 Vista Del Monte
Concord, CA 94520
(510) 692–2041
Fax (510) 692–2042

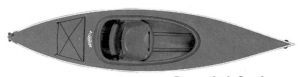

Perception's Caspia

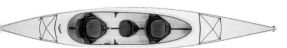

Perception's Jocassee

Mainstream Products
    182 Kayaker Way
    Easley, SC 29642
    (517) 323–2139

Necky Kayaks
    1100 Riverside Road
    Abbotsford, British Columbia
    V2S 7P1
    (604) 850–1206
    Fax (604) 850–3197

Old Town Canoe Company
    58 Middle Street
    Old Town, ME 04468
    (207) 827–5513
    Fax (207) 827–2779

Perception, Inc.
    P.O. Box 8002
    Easley, SC 29641
    (803) 859–7518
    Fax (803) 855–5995

Phoenix Poke Boats
    P.O. Box 109
    207 North Broadway
    Berea, KY 40403-0109
    (606) 986–2336
    Fax (606) 986–3277

Down the Yellowstone

Steve Chapple, burned out from living too long in the big city, moved back to his native Montana, took a few kayaking lessons, and then (with his wife and two sons) paddled the length of the Yellowstone River—at 671 miles the longest free-flowing river in the Lower 48. The adventure, full of colorful descriptions of the interesting personalities he met along the way, is chronicled in his fine book, *Kayaking the Full Moon* (New York: HarperCollins, 1993)

Prijon/Wildwasser Sport USA
    P.O. Box 4617
    Boulder, CO 80306
    (303) 444–2336
    Fax (303) 444–2375

Pygmy Boats
    P.O. Box 1529
    Port Townsend, WA 98368
    (360) 385–6143
    Fax (360) 379–9326

Seda Products
    926 Coolidge Avenue
    National City, CA 91950
    (619) 336–2444
    Fax (619) 336–2405

Swift Canoe & Kayak
    RR 1 Oxtongue Lake
    Dwight, Ontario P0A 1H0
    (705) 635–1167
    Fax (705) 635–9456

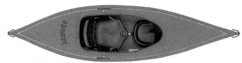

Perception's Keowee

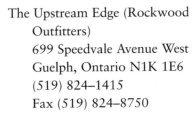

The Upstream Edge (Rockwood
    Outfitters)
    699 Speedvale Avenue West
    Guelph, Ontario N1K 1E6
    (519) 824–1415
    Fax (519) 824–8750

Tsunami
    13732 Bear Mountain Road
    Redding, CA 96003
    (916) 275–4313
    Fax (916) 275–3090

Valhalla Surf Ski Products
    4724 Renex Place
    San Diego, CA 92117
    (619) 569–1395
    Fax (619) 569–0295

Vermont Canoe Products
    RR 1, Box 353A
    Newport, VT 05855
    (800) 454–2307
    Fax (802) 754–2307

Walden Paddlers
    152 Commonwealth Avenue
    Concord, MA 01742
    (508) 371–3000

Wilderness Systems
    P.O. Box 4339
    Archdale, NC 27263
    (910) 434–7470
    Fax (910) 434–6912

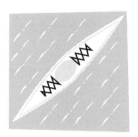

Chapter 6
Sea Kayaks

Sea kayaks are by far the most efficient and safest boats for self-propelled travel on large bodies of water. Many casual touring boats have a large storage capacity, but they are difficult to paddle under windy conditions and are dangerous for paddling in turbulent waters. Whitewater kayaks are stable in waves, but they do not track well and they offer little storage space. The sea kayak, on the other hand, is specifically made to handle these elements.

Sea Kayak Design

On open waters the ever-present forces are wind and waves, so a kayak that moves ahead efficiently and tracks well is essential. The ultimate goal of sea kayak design, then, is to reduce the adverse effects of wind and waves. The hull must also be large enough to carry your camping gear and equipment.

To improve the sea kayak's ability to move in a straight line (known as tracking), you need a long kayak with limited rocker (upturn). The limited rocker means that

more of the keel is in the water, thereby preventing the kayak from easily changing direction.

To keep the boat out of the wind, the height of a sea kayak deck is lowered, leaving just enough room ahead of the cockpit for knees and enough buoyancy in the bow for lifting above the waves. Reducing the deck's height to avoid the wind can go too far, however, to the point where the boat is easily capsized by waves.

Basic sea kayak designs reflect the conditions the boats are to be used in. Sea kayakers can often be heard to say that a particular model is of the "West Greenland style." These boats are stable, ocean-going craft that are predictable and easy to roll. They have rockered ends and a long, elegant bow. Their primary drawback is the lack of carrying capacity for gear, since they are streamlined to reduce wind resistance. The Nordkapp design is the premier example of the West Greenland Eskimo style of sea kayak and is used worldwide. (Nordkapp owners have their own organization:

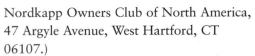

Nordkapp Owners Club of North America, 47 Argyle Avenue, West Hartford, CT 06107.)

Sea kayaks designed in England—following in the tradition of the West Greenland style—are generally noted for their remarkable rough-water performance. This is because they have evolved along the exposed coast of the British Isles, where tumultuous waves are the rule. These narrower kayaks have more rounded hulls, which allow the kayaker to more easily lean into the wave or to Eskimo roll the boat. The bow flare of these kayaks keeps them from burying their bows when surfing waves.

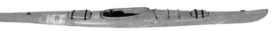

Dagger Canoe Co.'s Seeker

Kayaks designed in the Pacific Northwest, on the other hand, reflect the geographical conditions of hundreds of miles of protected waterways, where a kayaker is not exposed to the rigors of the open sea unless he or she chooses to paddle beyond the chain of islands. Boats designed for this

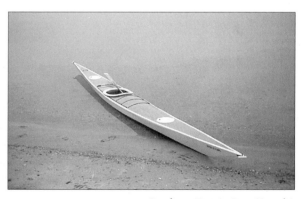

Recluse (Betsie Bay Kayak)

Instructional Videos

Among the excellent sea kayaking videos available are:
Performance Sea Kayaking: The Basics and Beyond
Sea Kayaking (Trailside Series)
Greenland Style Kayaking
You can get these videos from Great River Outfitters, 4180 Elizabeth Lake Road, Waterford, MI 48328; (248) 683–4770.

area are often large volume, with high peaked decks, large hatches, and roomy cockpits. These boats are very comfortable for long trips, have high initial stability, and can carry tremendous amounts of gear. Accordingly, they also have a high wind profile. Some of them are not well suited to rough seas, and they are usually more difficult to Eskimo roll.

Sea Kayak Features

If you're in the market for a sea kayak, take a close look at the following features before making your decision:

Hatches and Bulkheads

An important aspect of sea kayaks is the fitting of watertight storage compartments with bulkheads and hatches. With watertight bulkheads, no additional flotation is necessary. Various bulkhead arrangements are possible in a customized boat: for example, the front bulkhead can be moved to serve as a foot brace, increasing storage space but reducing cockpit volume. The rear bulkhead can likewise be moved flush with the cockpit rim to increase storage space.

Compass and Light

For safety reasons a compass is strongly recommended as a deck fitting. A compass light makes night paddling and navigation by chart after darkness easier.

Rudder

Rudders are commonly made an option on kayaks, though a few boats are designed to be used without them. Rudders generally make turning the boat easier. Some boaters disclaim rudders because they feel they are used as a crutch for poor technique, and because they are prone to failure in severe conditions or can inhibit landings and take-offs. However, the designs and materials of rudders have progressed in recent years and they are now accepted by most boaters.

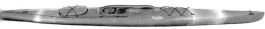

Dagger Canoe Co.'s Vesper

Retractable Skeg

A skeg is a fixed, rudderlike fin under the stern of the boat, and like a rudder, its purpose is to increase directional stability. The skeg blade is completely enclosed in a watertight box inside the kayak's rear compartment. This almost foolproof system adds a lot of versatility to kayaks. The question of rudders on sea kayaks has always been controversial, and the retractable skeg offers an alternative for those who are undecided.

Deck-fitted Bilge Pump

The deck-fitted bilge pump allows the paddler to begin emptying the kayak of water even if he or she has fallen out of the boat in deep water, and to continue by getting back into the boat and completing the pumping. For serious expeditions, the pump

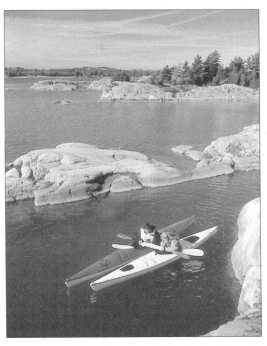

Caspian Sea (front) and North Sea Kayaks, (courtesy Swift Canoe & Kayak Co.)

has revolutionized deep-water rescues and provides an extra margin of safety. Different pump configurations are available. One is fitted on the deck behind the cockpit. Another is installed flush with the deck and has a detachable handle, which can be stowed under deck lines; the great advantages of this pump are its higher output and its easier accessibility, especially during self-rescues.

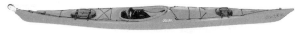

Dagger Canoe Co.'s Magellan

Finding the Right Boat

There has been a tendency of some U.S. designers to adopt more characteristics of the West Greenland style into their kayaks,

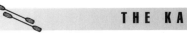
which has led to some narrowing of differences between that spare, rough-water style and the generally higher, roomier cut of American-designed boats. For kayakers who want to paddle along unprotected sections of coastline, the performance of the kayak in wind and waves should be the most significant factor in choosing a boat.

British Canoe Union Instruction

The premier British paddling association is the British Canoe Union, which sets safety standards and provides instruction. The BCU now offers sea kayaking courses in the U.S. through the following companies:

Atlantic Kayak Tours
   320 West Saugerties Road 7
   Saugerties, NY 12477
   (914) 246–2187

Great River Outfitters
   4180 Elizabeth Lake Road
   Waterford, MI 48328
   (248) 683–4770
   Fax: (248) 683–0306

Maine Island Kayak Company
   70 Luther Street
   Peaks Island, ME 04108
   (800) 796–2373

Sweetwater Kayaks
   5263 Ocean Boulevard, Siesta Key
   Sarasota, FL 34242
   (941) 346–1179

Trek & Trail
   P.O. Box 906
   222 Rittenhouse Avenue
   Batfield, MI 54814
   (800) 354–8735

In selecting a sea kayak, you'll go through the same basic steps that should be taken in contemplating any kayak purchase.

- Decide what kind of paddling you expect to do. Will you use your sea kayak in calm water most of the time? Or for extended coastal cruising? Or for open-water expeditions?
- Study a number of kayaks that appear to be suitable.
- Paddle the boat of your choice in as many different conditions as possible.
- Assess its performance in relation to hull shape and weight.
- Talk to experienced paddlers about their own boats.

When considering a purchase, keep in mind that all designs entail a compromise that balances one characteristic against another, and that the ultimate decision is yours alone. In addition to considering the type of sea kayaking you expect to do, take into account the amount of gear you will need to carry. As with other types of kayaks, try it out on the water before you buy.

Safety Gear for Sea Kayaking

Recommended safety equipment on a sea kayak includes the following. (See Chapter 15 for more details on safety gear.)

- Personal flotation device.
- Bilge pump.
- Compass.
- Flashing beacons, flares, and smoke devices.
- Whistle.
- Paddle float. This inflatable bag fits on the end of a kayak paddle for use as a stabilizing outrigger to aid a paddler in reentering the boat after a capsize.

- Sponsors. These inflatable pontoons will help stabilize the kayak as you scramble back aboard.
- VHF radio. It's the most effective emergency signaling device.
- EPIRB. An Emergency Position Indicating Radio Beacon is an emergency locator beacon that will send out an electronic call for help on frequencies monitored all over the world.
- Personal towline. This length of rope can be used to tow a boater in trouble.
- Sea anchor. It's essentially an underwater parachute used to avoid broaching in high winds and storm-tossed seas.
- Sea sock. This is a large bag that fits into the cockpit and is fitted over the cockpit coaming to limit the amount of water that can enter the boat.
- First-aid kit.
- Gloves.

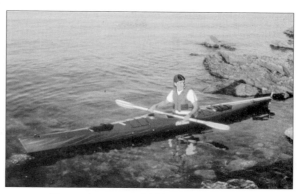

Heron (courtesy Old Town Canoe Co.)

- Nautical charts (large- and small-scale)
- Topographic maps (check for usefulness)
- Chart pack
- Compasses (deck compass and bearing compass)
- Watch (waterproof, with stopwatch; plus backup)
- Pencils and eraser
- Grease pencil with string attached
- Navigation notebook (preferably with waterproof paper)
- Highlight markers (two or three colors to mark charts and notes)
- Large flat ruler with string attached

Navigational Gear for Sea Kayaking

Navigational expert David Burch recommends the following:

Across the Atlantic

In 1956 a German named Hannes Lindemann crossed the Atlantic Ocean alone in a 17-foot Klepper folding kayak. It took him 72 days. His diet consisted mostly of evaporated milk and raw fish, but he allowed himself one can of beer a day.

Along the way, Lindemann encountered tremendous storms and was nearly capsized on several occasions by huge porpoises. His military surplus sextants were lost at sea, and he finished the trip by dead reckoning. He was the only kayaker ever to be featured on the cover of *Life* magazine. Amazingly enough, Lindemann may have found the journey a little anticlimactic: the previous year he had crossed the Atlantic in a 23-foot canoe.

An English translation of his book *Alone at Sea* is available from Western Folding Kayak Center, 6155 Mt. Aukum Road, Somerset, CA 95684; (530) 626–8647.

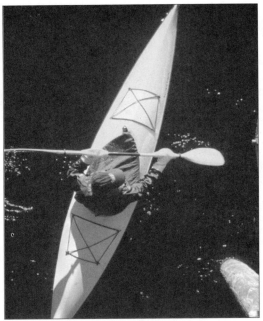

Walden Vision (courtesy Walden Paddlers, Inc.)

- Eyeglasses (if needed, plus backup)
- Sunglasses
- Pertinent sections of:
  Tide tables
  Current tables
  Coast Pilot or Sailing Directions
  Light list
  Special current references (if available)
  Tips from tour guides (if available)
- Marine weather services chart
- VHF radio plus waterproof bag
- List of VHF channels for marine operators
- Notes on VHF radio usage
- (Weather radio if no VHF available)
- Shortwave and AM radio receiver
- Binoculars
- Light for chart reading (spare bulbs and batteries)
- Some form of compass lighting (spare bulbs and batteries)

- Waterproof bag to hold navigational gear
- Heavy-duty rubber bands (to keep things organized)

Also useful is the GPS. Global Positioning System receivers are hand-held units that use satellites to locate your position.

Kayak Symposiums

During the year sea kayakers come together at symposiums and workshops to exchange ideas. Listed below are a number of the better-known ones. For information on dates and other details, contact the Trade Association of Paddlesports (12455 North Wauwatosa Road, Mequon, WI 53097; 414–242–5228) or the sources cited in the following list.

Advanced Coastal Kayaking Workshop. Contact: L.L. Bean, Inc., Freeport, ME 04033

Alaska Pacific University Kayak Symposium. Contact: Alaska Pacific University, 4101 University Drive, Anchorage, AK 99508

The Lure of Sea Kayaking

"The sea provides the unfamiliar, the unworn, and the unexpected. Sea kayaking gives a person the opportunity to venture on to a wild, unpredictable expanse in a craft that moves solely by the strength of their arm, directed by their experience and knowledge. Facing the challenge of the sea in this way causes a paddler to journey into the genuine unknown—the unknown and untried areas of his own soul."

—Derek C. Hutchinson
The Complete Book of Sea Kayaking

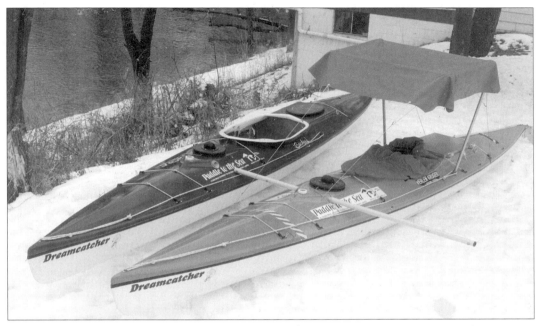

Two Dreamcatchers, with optional spray skirt, catamaran pole, and canopy to the right (courtesy Kruger Canoes)

Angel Island Festival & Regatta. Contact: Sea Trek Ocean Kayaking Center, Liberty Ship Way, Sausalito, CA 94965

Atlantic Coast Sea Kayaking Symposium. Contact: L.L. Bean, Inc., Freeport, ME 04033

East Coast Sea Kayaking Symposium (Charleston, South Carolina). Contact: Trade Association of Sea Kayaking, Box 84144, Seattle, WA 98124

Great Lakes Kayak Touring Symposium. Contact: Great River Outfitters, 4180 Elizabeth Lake Road, Waterford, MI 48238

Hornby Island Kayaker's Festival. Contact: Hornby Paddling Partners, RR 1, Hornby Island, British Columbia, V0R 1Z0

Inland Sea Kayaking Symposium. Contact: Trek & Trail, Box 906, Bayfield, WI 54814

Jersey Shore Sea Kayaking & Bay Canoeing Show. Contact: Ocean County De-

partment of Parks, Lakewood, NJ 08701

Mystic Sea Kayaking Symposium. Contact: Mystic Valley Sea Kayaking, 26 Williams Avenue, Mystic, CT 06355

West Coast Sea Kayaking Symposium. Contact: Trade Association of Sea Kayaking, Box 84144, Seattle, WA 98124

West Michigan Coastal Kayaking Symposium. Contact: Lumbertown Canoe & Kayak Specialties, 1822 Oake Avenue, North Muskegon, MI 49445

The Builders

Among the manufacturers of sea kayaks are Current Designs and Necky, and some of their boats are discussed here. You'll find statistical details on sea kayaks made by these and other manufacturers in the fact grids that follow this section.

Sources of Nautical Maps and Tide Charts

Eastern Distribution Branch
   U.S. Geological Survey
   604 South Pickett Street
   Alexandria, VA 22304

Western Distribution Branch
   U.S. Geological Survey
   Box 25286
   Federal Center
   Denver, CO 80225

Canada Map Office
   Surveys and Mapping Branch

Department of Energy, Mines, and Resources
   Ottawa, Ontario K1A 0E9

National Ocean Services
   Distribution Division (N/CG33)
   Riverdale, MD 20737

Captain's Nautical Supply
   1914 Fourth Avenue
   Seattle, WA 98101
   (800) 448–2278

Current Designs

Current Designs is a Canadian manufacturer based in Sidney, British Columbia, where it has been building boats since 1982. Its boats are distributed in the United States by We-no-nah Canoe in Winona, Minnesota.

When Brian Henry of Current Designs saw and paddled the 17-foot, 8-inch Caribou LXT, he was so impressed that he asked its designer, Barry Buchanan, if he would like Current Designs to produce his kayak. It is best described as a modified Greenland design with a narrow, hard-chine hull and a low deck profile. The hard-chine design offers high stability, while the narrow beam and low deck create a reduced wind profile and a sporty look. The 49-pound Caribou LXT features a clean deck arrangement with flush fiberglass hatches fore and

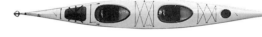

Current Designs/We-no-nah Canoe's Libra

aft. The seat comes with a comfortably padded back-band. The cockpit is molded with padded thigh braces shaped to fit a wide range of paddler sizes. Price: $2350 (fiberglass); $2850 (Kevlar).

The Gulfstream, named after the ocean current that joins North America and Europe, represents a union of effort through the collaboration of designers from both of these continents. British designer and paddler Derek Hutchinson teamed up with designer Brian Henry of Current Designs to develop this boat. Building on the strengths of Hutchinson's favorite kayak hull, the two men created the 17-foot Gulfstream to deliver a blend of British flair and performance with a North American influence and high-tech construction. Thanks to the technology of vacuum bagging, this kayak weighs only 50 pounds in fiberglass and 46

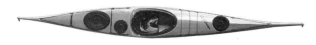

Current Designs/We-no-nah Canoe's Gulfstream

pounds in Kevlar. Features such as recessed deck fittings and perimeter lines are standard on the Gulfstream, as is a retractable skeg. Price: $2600–$3100.

The Expedition is Current Designs' response to demands for a high-performance kayak capable of carrying the loads necessary to sustain an expedition. At 18 feet, 10 inches long, with a narrow beam, the Expedition combines form and function in a hull that pivots and maneuvers easily. The Expedition increases efficiency by using its fish form to catch and run with swells. Its long waterline supports tracking, while a full bow contributes to a dry ride. Price: $2700–$3200.

The Solstice line also offers an expedition model, the Solstice GT (Grand

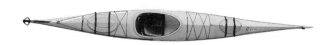

Current Designs/We-no-nah Canoe's Storm

Touring). The GT has a flared bow and stem and increased capacity in the deck, helping to give the paddler a dry ride. The cockpit is 31 inches long, affording easy entry and exit even for larger paddlers. The GT has a flush, large-access forward hatch and recessed deck fittings and perimeter safety lines. Price: $2600–$3100.

The 17-foot Storm is Current Design's first roto-molded plastic kayak, and it's designed to handle abuse. The linear polyethylene hull provides a combination of strength, stiffness, and impact resistance. Ultraviolet stabilizers added to the plastic help prevent breakdown caused by the sun. The Storm's recessed deck fittings accommodate a clean deck-rigging system with full

Current Designs/We-no-nah Canoe's Libra profile

Across the Pacific

"When I said that I was planning to paddle across 2,200 miles of open ocean in a twenty-foot kayak, people looked at me as though I had told them I was going to commit suicide," said Ed Gillet of his 63-day paddle across the Pacific from Monterey, California, to Hawaii.

Gillet came well-prepared for the journey, with a reverse osmosis pump to convert saltwater to freshwater, a VHF radio to contact passing ships, an emergency radio beacon to alert aircraft, flares, signal mirrors, a strobelight, and a radar reflector. His boat had a wooden floor so he could sleep a few inches above the water sloshing about inside. Pontoons could be deployed to allow him to move about the boat without fear of capsizing, and a sailor's harness tethered him to the kayak.

The "cruise" was not without its hardships. After only a few days, Gillet's body was covered with saltwater sores, and within a week, his hands were so chapped he had to take painkillers. Next he met relentless storms. Then he was becalmed, a thousand miles from land. It got worse: He ran out of food and started eating his toothpaste.

When Gillet finally plowed his bow into the sands of Maui, his legs collapsed beneath him. A local beach bum approached and asked where he had come from. When Gillet told him California, he whistled, "That's a long way. Must've taken you two or three days, huh?"

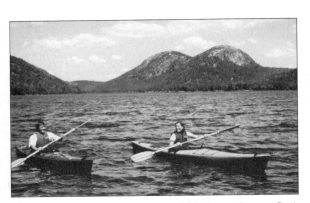

Egret (courtesy Old Town Canoe Co.)

perimeter deck lines. The rudder mounting and blade locator slot are molded into the rear deck, eliminating potential leaks from screws. Price: $1400.

The Squall is the little (16 feet, 6 inches) sister of the Storm, scaled down for the smaller paddler or for someone wanting a slimmer, tighter-fitting craft with all of the features and details of the Storm. Price: $1400.

Necky

Necky Kayaks, a Canadian company based in Abbotsford, British Columbia, has been building touring boats since 1983. It offers a wide range of sea kayaks in polyethylene, fiberglass, and Kevlar.

One of Necky's best-known lines is the Looksha series, which consists of five double hard-chined models. The waterline of these boats is evenly rockered, and the volume distribution resembles a torpedo, with slightly more room in the bow. This gives better handling in rough conditions.

The Looksha II is an all-around boat designed with a highly rockered, fast-turning hull. It is 20 feet long and 20 inches wide, and available in fiberglass or Kevlar. Price: $2300–$2700.

The Looksha III, more stable than the Looksha II, is available with an adjustable skeg or rudder. It is 19 feet, 6 inches long and 21 inches wide, and also is available in fiberglass or Kevlar. Price: $2300–$2700.

The Looksha IV is designed as an all-around touring kayak, with enough stability for the recreational paddler but playful enough for the skillful kayaker. The double chine allows a relatively small wetted surface with good stability through all positions, while increasing stability during an extreme lean. It is 17 feet long, and available in superlinear polymer, fiberglass, or Kevlar. Price: $1250–$2600.

Popular Sea Kayaking Destinations

There are countless touring possibilities, but here are a few good areas in North America to whet your appetite:

Prince William Sound, Alaska
Kodiak Island, Alaska
Glacier Bay, Alaska
Queen Charlotte Islands, British Columbia
Vancouver Island, British Columbia
San Juan Islands, Washington
Monterey Bay National Marine Sanctuary, California
Sea of Cortez, Mexico
Magdelena Bay, Mexico
Florida Keys
Everglades National Park, Florida
Coast of North and South Carolina
Lake Superior, Michigan
Boundary Waters Canoe Area, Minnesota
Coast of Maine

Also offered by Necky is the lower-volume Looksha IVS for the lighter paddler. The overall volume of this 16-foot, 6-inch boat is decreased, as is the length, weight, and width. Available in fiberglass or Kevlar. Price: $2200–$2600.

The 14-foot, 4-inch Looksha Sport was designed for fast turning, especially on a lean, but also for straight tracking when on an even keel. It's a good boat for playing in rock gardens, surf, mangrove swamps, or tight rivers. Available in polymer, fiberglass, or Kevlar, with optional rudder or skeg. Price: $650–$2400.

The Arluk I, also 18 feet long, is a mid-size touring boat with a buoyant bow that helps it ride over waves and avoid diving in following seas. Price: $2200–$2600.

The length of the Arluk III (16 feet) makes it more portable and easier to turn. Beginning paddlers will appreciate its stability and maneuverability on short trips, and even in demanding water. Price: $2200–$2600.

The Tesla model handles similarly to the Arluk but is more stable, has a higher cargo capacity, and is suited for paddlers who need more legroom. The 17-foot Tesla is a good candidate for extended expeditions. Price: $2100 (fiberglass); $2500 (Kevlar).

Necky offers a number of tandem models. The polyethylene Amaruk provides four flotation compartments, contributing to easier self-rescue. Aluminum tubing on the bottom of the hull acts as a stiffener. Price: $1550.

The tandem Tofino is a high-volume boat that provides a third bulkhead to stop water from sloshing the length of the boat and to allow separate rescue from either

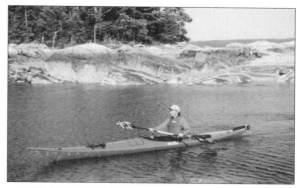

Millennium 174 (courtesy Old Town Canoe Co.)

paddling position. The fish-form design contributes to good handling in rough conditions. Price: $2750 (fiberglass); $3150 (Kevlar).

The 22-foot-long Nootka is a sporty tandem created to be a fast sea-touring model with low windage and enough room for gear. Paddling compartments are separated by a bulkhead to facilitate rescues. A rudder is standard. Kevlar only. Price: $3350.

Sea Kayak Manufacturers

Ainsworth
P.O. Box 207
Norwich, VT 05055
(802) 649–2952
Fax (802) 649–2254

Baldwin Boat Company
RR 2, Box 268
Orrington, ME 04474
(207) 825–4439

Baltic Kayaks
330 McKinley Terrace
Centerport, NY 11721
(516) 673–4662
Fax (516) 673–8352

Classic Sea Journeys

Here are a couple of books every sea kayaker should have in their library, just for inspiration:

Seekers of the Horizon, edited by Will Nordby (The Globe Pequot Press, 1989): a collection of stories from around the world about paddling journeys, varying in length from day trips to an 8,000-mile solo expedition.

The Hidden Coast, by Joel W. Rogers (Seattle: Alaska Northwest Books, 1991): a beautiful coffee-table book, full of stunning photography, covering the western coastline from Alaska to Mexico.

Betsie Bay Kayak
 P.O. Box 1706
 Frankfort, MI 49635
 (616) 352–7774

Boreal Design
 108 Amsterdam
 Industrial Park
 St. Augustin, Quebec G3A 1V9
 (418) 878–3099
 Fax (418) 878–3459

Cal-Tek Engineering
 36 Riverside Drive
 Kingston, MA 02364
 [781] 585–5666

Dagger Canoe Co's Meridian

Current Designs
 10124 McDonald Park Road
 Sidney, British Columbia V8L 5X8
 (250) 655–1822
 Fax (250) 655–1596
 E-mail: info@cdkayak.com
 Web: http://www.cdkayak.com

Dagger Canoe Company
 P.O. Box 1500
 Harriman, TN 37748
 (423) 882–0404
 Fax (423) 882–8153

Easy Rider Canoe & Kayak Company
 P.O. Box 88108
 Seattle, WA 98138
 (425) 228–3633
 Fax (425) 277–8778

Eddyline Kayaks
 1344 Ashten Road
 Burlington, WA 98233
 (360) 757–2300

Englehart Products Inc. (EPI)
 P.O. Box 377
 Newbury, OH 44065
 (216) 564–5565
 Fax (216) 564–5515

Euro Kayaks/TG Canoe Livery
 P.O. Box 177
 Martindale, TX 78655
 (512) 353–3946
 Fax (512) 353–3947

Glenwa
P.O. Box 3134
Gardena, CA 90247
(310) 327–9216
Fax (310) 327–8952
E-mail: cobrakayaks@worldnet.att.net
Web: http://www.cobrakayaks.com

Dagger Canoe Co.'s Edisto

Great Canadian Canoe Company
64 Worcester Providence Turnpike
Sutton, MA 01590
(508) 865–0010
Fax (508) 865–5220

Hop On Top Kayaks
P.O. Box 139
Jamestown, RI 02835
(401) 423–1815
Fax (401) 423–1815

Hydra Kayaks
5061 South National Drive
Knoxville, TN 37914
(800) 537–8888
Fax (305) 836–1296

Island Innovations
738 Selkirk Avenue
Victoria, British Columbia V9A 2T5
(250) 388–7466

Janautica/Splashdance
Highway 85 South
Niceville, FL 32578
(850) 678–1637
Fax (850) 678–1637
Web: http://www.splashdance.com

Kiwi Kayak Company
2454 Vista Del Monte
Concord, CA 94520
(510) 692–2041
Fax (510) 692–2042

Finding Your Way

The premier reference for matters navigational is *Fundamentals of Kayak Navigation,* by David Burch (The Globe Pequot Press, 1993). No serious sea kayaker should be without it.

Other excellent navigation books you could add to your library are:

The Essential Wilderness Navigator, by David Seidman (Camden, Maine: International Marine, 1995)

Boat Navigation for the Rest of Us: Finding Your Way by Eye and Electronics, by Bill Brogdon (International Marine, 1995)

Celestial Navigation for Yachtsmen (revised edition), by Mary Blewitt, edited by Thomas C. Bergel (International Marine, 1996)

Emergency Navigation: Pathfinding Techniques for the Inquisitive and Prudent Mariner, by David Burch (International Marine, 1989)

The Practical Pilot: Coastal Navigation by Eye, Intuition, and Common Sense, by Leonard Eyges (International Marine, 1989)

Tide Tables

Tide tables and tide current tables are a necessity in areas affected by tides, where you need to know the velocities of ebb and flow currents and information on rotary currents. The latest National Oceanic and Atmospheric Administration tide tables (four volumes, covering various geographical areas around the world) and tidal current tables (two volumes, one for the Atlantic coast of North America and the other for the Pacific coast of North America) are available from International Marine, P.O. Box 182607, Columbus, OH 43218; (800) 262–4729.

Kruger Canoes
  2906 Meister Lane
  Lansing, MI 48906
  (517) 323–2139

Mainstream Products
  182 Kayaker Way
  Easley, SC 29642
  (517) 323–2139

Mariner Kayaks
  2134 Westlake Avenue North
  Seattle, WA 98109
  (206) 284–8404
  Fax (206) 284–6046

Necky Kayaks
  1100 Riverside Road
  Abbotsford, British Columbia
  V2S 7P1
  (604) 850–1206
  Fax (604) 850–3197

Nomad Kayaks
  4918 boul. Rive Sud
  Levis, Quebec G6W 5N6
  (418) 838–0338
  Fax (418) 838–0801

Northwest Kayaks
  15145 NE 90th Street
  Redmond, WA 98052
  (425) 869–1107
  Fax (425) 869–9014

Ocean Kayak
  P.O. Box 5003
  Ferndale, WA 98248
  (800) 852–9257
  Fax (360) 366–2628

Old Town Canoe Company
  58 Middle Street
  Old Town, ME 04468
  (207) 827–5513
  Fax (207) 827–2779

Pacific Water Sports
  16055 Pacific Highway South
  Seattle, WA 98188
  (206) 246–9385
  Fax (206) 439–9040

P & H Designs/Impex International
  1107 Station Road, Unit 1
  Bellport, NY 11713
  (516) 286–1988
  Fax (516) 286–1952

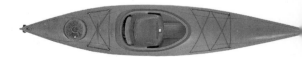

Perception's Acadia

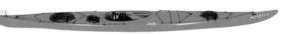

Dagger Canoe Co.'s Apostle

Perception, Inc.
P.O. Box 8002
Easley, SC 29641
(803) 859–7518
Fax (803) 855–5995

Phoenix Poke Boats
P.O. Box 109
207 North Broadway
Berea, KY 40403-0109
(606) 986–2336
Fax (606) 986–3277

Prijon/Wildwasser Sport USA
P.O. Box 4617
Boulder, CO 80306
(303) 444–2336
Fax (303) 444–2375

Pyranha/Impex International
1107 Station Road
Bellport, NY 11713
(516) 286–1988
Fax (516) 286–1952

Rainforest Designs
P.O. Box 91
Maple Ridge, British Columbia
V0M 1B0
(604) 467–9932
Fax (604) 467–8890

Seaward Kayaks
RR 1, Site 16
Summerland, British Columbia
V0H 1Z0
(800) 595–9755
Fax (250) 494–5200

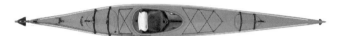

Perception's Chinook NW

Seda Products
926 Coolidge Avenue
National City, CA 91950
(619) 336–2444
Fax (619) 336–2405

Southern Exposure Sea Kayaks
P.O. Box 4530
Tequesta, FL 33469
(561) 575–4530
Fax (561) 744–9371

Profile: Don Starkell

Don Starkell is a man possessed. In 1980, he canoed the 12,281 miles from Winnipeg to the mouth of the Amazon, a journey chronicled in his book *Paddle to the Amazon: The Ultimate 12,000-Mile Canoe Adventure* (Toronto: McCleland & Stewart, 1995).

In 1990, at the age of 57, he began, by kayak, the 3,200-mile journey from Hudson Bay through the Northwest Passage. The trek took three summers, and the diary of that trip from Churchill, Manitoba, north and then west to Tuktoyaktuk, near Alaska, is published as *Paddle to the Arctic* (also published by McCleland & Stewart in 1995). It's a fascinating read, full of drama as Starkell races against the winter to finish the journey—and to save his life.

Weather Watching

For the serious sea kayaker, highly recommended is the new interactive computer program for recognizing and dealing with bad weather at sea, Starpath Weather Trainer. The program, by David Burch, is available from International Marine, P.O. Box 182607, Columbus, OH 43218; (800) 262–4729.

Wilderness System's Alto

Superior Kayaks
P.O. Box 355
Whitelaw, WI 54247
(920) 732–3784
E-mail: kayaks@aol.com

Tsunami
13732 Bear Mountain Road
Redding, CA 96003
(916) 275–4313
Fax (916) 275–3090

Valley Canoe Products/Great River Outfitters
4180 Elizabeth Lake Road
Waterford, MI 48328
(248) 683–4770
Fax (248) 683–0306

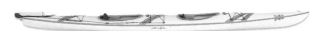

Wilderness System's Echo

Vermont Canoe Products
RR 1, Box 353A
Newport, VT 05855
(800) 454–2307
Fax (802) 754–2307

Swift Canoe & Kayak
RR 1 Oxtongue Lake
Dwight, Ontario P0A 1H0
(705) 635–1167

Walden Paddlers
152 Commonwealth Avenue
Concord, MA 01742
(508) 371–3000

The Upstream Edge (Rockwood Outfitters)
699 Speedvale Avenue West
Guelph, Ontario N1K 1E6
(519) 824–1415
Fax (519) 824–8750

West Side Boat Shop
7661 Tanawanda Creek Road
Lockport, NY 14094
(716) 434–5755

Trent Canoe & Kayak
2350 Haines Road
Bldg. 28
Mississauga, Ontario L4Y 1Y6
(905) 273–9075
Fax (905) 275–3090

Wilderness System's Sealution II

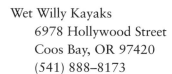 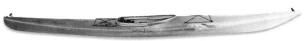
Wet Willy Kayaks
6978 Hollywood Street
Coos Bay, OR 97420
(541) 888–8173

Wilderness System's Piccolo

Wilderness Systems
P.O. Box 4339
Archdale, NC 27263
(910) 434–7470
Fax (910) 434–6912

Woodstrip Watercraft Company
1818 Swamp Pike
Gilbertsville, PA 19525
(610) 326–9282

Wilderness System's Sea Two

Good Reads: Sea Kayaking

The Complete Book of Sea Kayaking, by Derek C. Hutchinson (The Globe Pequot Press, 1995)

Sea Kayaking: A Manual for Long-Distance Touring (second edition), by John Dowd (Seattle: University of Washington Press, 1997)

Derek C. Hutchinson's Guide to Expedition Kayaking on Sea and Open Water, by Derek C. Hutchinson (The Globe Pequot Press, 1999)

Nigel Foster's Sea Kayaking, by Nigel Foster (The Globe Pequot Press, 1997)

The Coastal Kayaker's Manual: A Complete Guide to Skills, Gear, and Sea Sense, by Randel Washburne (The Globe Pequot Press, 1998)

Sea Kayaking Basics, by David Harrison (New York: Hearst Marine Books, 1993)

The Essential Sea Kayaker: A Complete Course for the Open Water Paddler, by David Seidman (Camden, Maine: Ragged Mountain Press, 1992)

Sea Kayaks

The following grids present details on the lineup of sea kayaks offered by selected manufacturers. See above for the addresses and phone numbers of these and other manufacturers. For information on paddles, see Chapter 3. For information on spray skirts, life jackets, and other accessories, see Chapter 14.

Manufacturer/model	Length (feet)	Width (inches)	Weight (pounds)	Material
Baldwin (1966)				
Anchovy Series	13'2"	24	28-40*	fiberglass or Kevlar
Atlantic Series (including tandem)	17'	24	32-56*	fiberglass or Kevlar
Falcon Series	17'	24	24-44*	fiberglass or Kevlar
Baltic (1980)				
Argo Series (tandem)	17'9", 20'3"	26½, 27½	72-79	fiberglass
Mari Series	16'9"	22½	48-49*	fiberglass
Betsie Bay (1985)				
Idun	16'	20½'	35	wood
Manitou	17'10"	22	40	wood
Recluse	19'	20½	40	wood straight with rise at ends
Valkyrie	17'	21	38	wood
Boreal (1991)				
Alvik	17'	23	44-50*	fiberglass or Kevlar
Beluga (tandem)	21'	28½	70-78*	fiberglass or Kevlar
Minganie (tandem)	21'10"	30	84-95*	fiberglass or Kevlar
Narwhal	16'	24½	42-48*	fiberglass or Kevlar
Saguenay	18'	24	48-54*	fiberglass or Kevlar
Cal-Tek (1971)				
Caspian-Seal	16'6"	24	35	proprietary lay-up
Greenland	15'3"	24	32	proprietary lay-up
Harbor-Seal	16'6"	26	45	proprietary lay-up
Current Designs (1982)				
Breeze	13'6"	25	55	polyethylene
Caribou LXT	17'8"	21¾	41-49*	fiberglass or Kevlar
Expedition	18'10"	22¼	50-56*	fiberglass or Kevlar
Gulfstream	17'	24	46-52*	fiberglass or Kevlar
Libra Series (including tandem)	22'8", 22'9"	30, 31½	84-92*	fiberglass or Kevlar
Pachena	14'	25¼	42-50*	fiberglass or Kevlar
Slipstream	16'	21¼	41-49*	fiberglass or Kevlar
Solstice Series	17'6"	22¼-24½	50-55*	fiberglass or Kevlar
Speedster	19'11"	25	28-35	fiberglass or Kevlar
Squall	16'6"	22¼	61	polyethylene
Storm	17'	24	64	polyethylene
Dagger (1988)				
Apostle	17'	23½	68	polyethylene
Atlantis	17'3"	23	66	polyethylene
Edisto Expedition	14'6"	24½	55	polyethylene
Magellan	16'6"	22½	62	polyethylene
Meridian	16'	22	46-54*	fiberglass or Kevlar
Seeker Expedition	16'	23½	60	polyethylene
Sitka	17'10"	22	52-60*	fiberglass or Kevlar
Vesper Expedition	13'10"	24	57	polyethylene
Easy Rider (1970)				
Beluga Series (tandem)	16'8", 18'	32	65-78*	fiberglass or Kevlar
Dolphin Series	14'9"	24¼	29-45*	fiberglass or Kevlar
Eskimo Series (including tandem)	15'-22'6"	24½-30½	40-98*	fiberglass or Kevlar
Sea Eagle Series (tandem)	18'6", 19'	33	65-85*	fiberglass or Kevlar
Sea Hawk Series	17'	25¼	38-56*	fiberglass or Kevlar
Tatoosh (tandem)	16'8"	32	55-68*	fiberglass or Kevlar
Eddyline (1971)				
Falcon Series	16', 18'	20½, 21	40-56*	fiberglass or Kevlar
Merlin Series	13'6", 15'	23	45-52*	proprietary lay-up
Raven	16'9"	22	48-56*	fiberglass or Kevlar
Whisper (tandem)	19'	30	70-85*	fiberglass or Kevlar
Wind Dancer	17'	24	52-60*	fiberglass or Kevlar

Keel	Bottom	Sides	Price (dollars)
straight	shallow V	tumblehome	1100-1600*
straight	shallow V	tumblehome	1200-2000*
straight	shallow arch	flared	1200-2000*
straight with rise at ends	deep V or shallow arch	flared	1400-1500
straight with rise at ends	shallow arch	flared	1100-1350*
straight with rise at ends	shallow V	flared	3000
straight with rise at ends	shallow V	flared	3000
	shallow V	flared	3000
	shallow V	flared	3000
straight with rise at ends	shallow V	straight	1950-2250*
straight with rise at ends	shallow V	straight	2600-3100*
straight with rise at ends	shallow V	straight	2900-3400*
straight with rise at ends	shallow V	straight	1800-2100*
straight with rise at ends	rounded V	straight	2050-2350*
straight with rise at ends	shallow V	flared	1300
straight with rise at ends	shallow V	flared	1400
straight with rise at ends	shallow V	flared	1400
straight with rise at ends	shallow V	flared	850
straight with rise at ends	shallow V	flared	2350-2850*
straight with rise at ends	rounded V	flared	2700-3200*
straight with rise at ends	shallow V	flared	2600-3100*
straight with rise at ends	shallow V	flared	3000-4200*
straight with rise at ends	shallow V	flared	1850-2350*
straight with rise at ends	shallow V	straight	2600-3100*
straight with rise at ends	shallow V	flared	2400-3100*
straight with rise at ends	rounded V	flared	2700-3200
straight with rise at ends	shallow V	flared	1400
straight with rise at ends	shallow V	flared	1400
moderate rocker	shallow arch	flared	1150
straight with rise at ends	shallow arch	flared	1300
moderate rocker	shallow arch	flared	850
straight with rise at ends	shallow arch	flared	1150
straight with rise at ends	shallow arch	flared	2100-2500*
moderate rocker	shallow arch	flared	1050
straight with rise at ends	shallow arch	flared	2350-2650*
moderate rocker	shallow arch	flared	800
straight with rise at ends	shallow arch	flared	2400-3700*
straight with rise at ends	shallow arch	flared	1100-2200*
straight with rise at ends	shallow arch	flared	2700-6500*
straight with rise at ends	shallow V	flared	2500-3900*
straight with rise at ends	shallow V	flared	1350-2900*
straight with rise at ends	shallow V	flared	2500-3400*
extreme rocker	deep V	flared	2300-2500
extreme rocker	shallow V	flared	1500-1700
moderate rocker	shallow arch	flared	2450
moderate rocker	shallow arch	flared	3150
moderate rocker	shallow arch	flared	2500

Manufacturer/model	Length (feet)	Width (inches)	Weight (pounds)	Material
Englehart (1988)				
Epitour	14'	25	38	polyethylene
Episea (designed for women)	14'2"	20½	38	polyethylene
Euro (1986)				
Traveller K-1	14'1"	24¾	48	polyethylene
Traveller K-2 (tandem)	16'5"	29½	75	polyethylene
Glenwa (1992)				
Cobra Tourer	18'	28	49	polyethylene
Great Canadian (1972)				
River Runner R5 XL	14'	24	46	polyethylene
Sojourn	16'9"	24	58	fiberglass
Hop On Top (1995)				
16' HopOnTop	16'	27	39-45*	fiberglass or Kevlar
18' HopOnTop	18'3"	24	40-48*	fiberglass or Kevlar
Hydra (1992)				
Horizon	13'6"	23	55	polyethylene
Sea Runner XL	17'1"	24	65	polyethylene
Sea Twin (tandem)	18'2"	29	95	polyethylene
Sea Venture	16'2"	23	60	polyethylene
Solo	17'1"	22½	60	polyethylene
Island Innovations (1995)				
Triak	18'	21	95	fiberglass
Janautica/Splashdance (1983)				
Alaska	15'4"	23	39	fiberglass
Anadyr	17'5"	21	50	fiberglass
Haiti-tandem	17'8"	31	70	fiberglass
Samon	14'9"	25	44	fiberglass
Victoria	14'3"	26	36	fiberglass
Kiwi (1988)				
Lobo Gato	9'2"	28	40	polyethylene
Mark 4 (tandem)	13'6"	28	40	polyethylene
Mark Twain (tandem)	13'6"	29	61	polyethylene
Kruger (1971)				
Dreamcatcher	17'2"	28	79	Kevlar
Mainstream (1980)				
Tango	12'	34	52	polyethylene
Mariner (1980)				
Coaster	13'5"	23	35-40*	proprietary lay-up or Kevlar
Elan	16'2"	21½	34-44*	proprietary lay-up, Kevlar, or graphite
Escape Series	16'7"	24½	46-56*	proprietary lay-up or Kevlar
Express Series	16'	22½	42-53*	proprietary lay-up or Kevlar
Mariner MAX Series	17'	23½	45-55*	proprietary lay-up or Kevlar
Mariner II Series	17'11"	21½	40-55*	proprietary lay-up, Kevlar, or graphite
Mariner XL Series	17'1"	23½	44-54*	proprietary lay-up or Kevlar
Mega (1992)				
Diamente	16'6"	22¾	48	proprietary lay-up

Keel	Bottom	Sides	Price (dollars)
straight	shallow V	flared	600
straight	shallow arch	flared	600
straight	shallow arch	flared	850-1000*
straight	shallow arch	flared	1150-1300*
straight with rise at ends	shallow arch	straight	785
moderate rocker	shallow arch	flared	650
straight with rise at ends	shallow V	flared	1800
moderate rocker	shallow V	flared	1700-2100*
straight with rise at ends	rounded V	flared	1900-2300*
straight with rise at ends	shallow arch	flared	800
straight with rise at ends	shallow V	flared	1250
straight with rise at ends	shallow arch	flared	1450
moderate rocker	rounded V	flared	950
straight with rise at ends	shallow V	flared	950
straight with rise at ends	shallow arch	flared	4400
straight with rise at ends	shallow arch	tumblehome	1400
straight with rise at ends	rounded V	tumblehome	1500
straight with rise at ends	shallow arch	straight	2000
straight with rise at ends	flat	straight	1400
straight with rise at ends	shallow arch	tumblehome	1250
straight with rise at ends	shallow V	straight	1050
straight with rise at ends	shallow V	straight	1400
straight with rise at ends	shallow V	straight	650
straight with rise at ends	shallow arch	flared	3800
moderate rocker	shallow arch	straight	500
moderate rocker	shallow V	flared	2200-2600*
straight with rise at ends	shallow V	flared	2350-3100*
straight with rise at ends	shallow V	flared	2400-2800*
straight with rise at ends	shallow V	flared	2350-2800*
straight with rise at ends	shallow V	flared	2450-3200*
straight with rise at ends	shallow V	flared	2450-3200*
straight with rise at ends	shallow arch	flared	2350-2750*
straight with rise at ends	rounded V	flared	2300

Manufacturer/model	Length (feet)	Width (inches)	Weight (pounds)	Material
Mega Continued				
Peridot	15'	22	45	proprietary lay-up
Seasure	17'6"	23	50	proprietary lay-up
Necky (1983)				
Alsek	14'	24½	47-57*	fiberglass (chopper gun) or polyethylene
Amaruk (tandem)	19'	29	80	polyethylene
Arluk Series	18', 19'	21, 22	45-55*	fiberglass (chopper gun) or polyethylene
Kyook Series	15'	25	57-60*	polyethylene
Looksha Series	14'4", 17', 20'	20-23	43-60*	fiberglass (chopper gun), Kevlar, or polyethylene
Narpa	16'5"	24	60	polyethylene
Nootka (tandem)	22'	20	85	Kevlar
Pinta	17'4"	28	50-60*	fiberglass (chopper gun) or Kevlar
Santa Cruze (tandem)	13'	31	60	polyethylene
Tesla	17'	24	45-55*	fiberglass (chopper gun) or Kevlar
Tofino (tandem)	20'	31½	80-95*	fiberglass (chopper gun) or Kevlar
Tornak	15'6"	24	55-65*	fiberglass (chopper gun), Kevlar, or polyethylene
Nomad (1986)				
Exocet	17'4"	20½	45-50*	fiberglass or proprietary lay-up
Tango (tandem)	22'	28	78-84*	fiberglass or proprietary lay-up
Vagabond	16'9"	24½	43-48*	fiberglass or proprietary lay-up
Northwest (1979)				
Cadence Series	16'11"	23½	51-56*	fiberglass or Kevlar
Discover Series	17'11"	22	57-58*	fiberglass or Kevlar
Esprit	16'4"	23	47-52*	fiberglass or Kevlar
Photon Series	8'3", 8'7"	23, 23¾	26-38*	fiberglass, Kevlar, or polyethylene
Pursuit Series	16'10"-17'6"	22-23	54-65*	fiberglass, Kevlar, or polyethylene
Seascape Series (tandem)	18'4"-21'1"	30	80-105*	fiberglass or Kevlar
Sportee Series	13'6"	22½-23	45-53*	fiberglass, Kevlar, or polyethylene
Ocean (1971)				
Zest Two (tandem)	16'	32	68	polyethylene
Old Town (1898)				
Egret Series	14'6"	24½	54-57*	polyethylene
Heron	16'1"	24½	59	polyethylene
Millenium Series	17'4", 16'	22½-23	56-60*	polyethylene
P & H Designs (1972)				
Capella	17'	21½	52-57*	fiberglass or polyethylene
Orion	17'	24	55	fiberglass
Outlander	16'	24	52	fiberglass
Sirius Series	17'	20½	52-57*	fiberglass
Pacific Water Sports (1972)				
Avocet Series	16'	23	53-55*	fiberglass
Intrepid Series	17'6"	23	51-52*	fiberglass
Osprey Series	17'6"	23	54-56*	fiberglass
Sea Otter Series	16'4"	25	52-55*	fiberglass
Seal	18'	21	52	fiberglass
Shookumchuck Series (tandem)	21'	30	53-55*	fiberglass
TBird Series	17'6"	27½	68	fiberglass
Thunderbird Series	17'6"	27½	65-68*	fiberglass
Wigeon	14'3"	21½	42	fiberglass

Keel	Bottom	Sides	Price (dollars)
straight with rise at ends	rounded V	flared	2300
straight with rise at ends	rounded V	flared	2300
straight with rise at ends	shallow V	flared	1100-1400*
straight with rise at ends	shallow V	flared	1550
straight with rise at ends	shallow V	flared	2200-2600*
straight with rise at ends	shallow V	flared	700-1250*
straight with rise at ends	shallow V	flared	650-2700*
straight with rise at ends	shallow V	flared	1300
straight with rise at ends	shallow V	flared	3350
straight with rise at ends	shallow V	flared	2300-2800*
straight with rise at ends	shallow V	flared	800
straight with rise at ends	shallow V	flared	2100-2500*
straight with rise at ends	shallow V	flared	2750-3150*
straight with rise at ends	shallow V	flared	1250-2500*
straight with rise at ends	deep V	straight	1850-2250*
straight with rise at ends	shallow arch	tumblehome	2550-2950*
moderate rocker ends	shallow arch	tumblehome	1850-2250*
moderate rocker	shallow V	flared	2300-2800*
moderate rocker	shallow V	flared	2450-2900*
moderate rocker	shallow V	flared	2300-2700*
extreme rocker	flat	straight	850-1150*
moderate rocker	shallow V	flared	2300-2700*
moderate rocker	shallow V	flared	2800-4200*
moderate rocker	shallow V	flared	900-2350*
moderate rocker	deep V	straight	650-800*
straight with rise at ends	shallow arch	straight	650-750*
straight with rise at ends	shallow arch	straight	900
straight with rise at ends	shallow arch	flared	750-900*
straight with rise at ends	shallow V	flared	1100-1500*
straight with rise at ends	shallow V	flared	1200
straight with rise at ends	shallow V	flared	1100
straight with rise at ends	shallow V	flared	1100-1500*
straight with rise at ends	rounded V	straight	2300-2450*
straight with rise at ends	rounded V	straight	2300-2450*
straight with rise at ends	rounded V	straight	2350-2500*
straight with rise at ends	rounded V	straight	2300
straight with rise at ends	shallow arch	straight	2300
straight with rise at ends	rounded V	straight	3300
straight with rise at ends	rounded V	straight	2700
straight with rise at ends	rounded V	straight	2550-2700*
straight with rise at ends	flat	straight	1650

Manufacturer/model	Length (feet)	Width (inches)	Weight (pounds)	Material
Perception (1975)				
Aquaterra Acadia	12'4"	27	65	polyethylene
Aquaterra Chinook	16'1"	24	65	polyethylene
Aquaterra Scimitar	15'2"	23	64	polyethylene
Aquaterra Sea Lion Series	16'8", 17'2"**	22, 22½	57-62*	fiberglass, Kevlar, or polyethylene
Aquaterra Spectrum Series	13'5", 14'4"	24¾- 25¼	53-61*	polyethylene
Aquaterra Umiak	12'	21	35	polyethylene
Shadow	16'8"	22	62	polyethylene
Phoenix Poke Boats (1973)				
Brown Pelican	14'5"	27	26-32*	proprietary lay-up or Kevlar
Isere	14'9"	24	24-29*	proprietary lay-up or Kevlar
Vagabond K2 (tandem)	16'5"	29	40-46*	proprietary lay-up or Kevlar
Prijon (1985)				
Odyssee	16'1"	26	75	polyethylene
Seayak Expedition	16'1"	24	55	polyethylene
Yukon Tour	14'5"	25	44	polyethylene
Pyranha (1974)				
Orca Duo (tandem)	16'	24	65	polyethylene
Orca Expedition	15'	22	45	polyethylene
Rainforest Designs (1990)				
Nimbus Cygnet	14'9"	23	40-46*	fiberglass or Kevlar
Nimbus Horizon	16'3"	23½	45-53*	fiberglass or Kevlar
Nimbus Hyak (tandem)	19'3"	28	80-95*	fiberglass or Kevlar
Nimbus Kanaka (tandem)	18'3"	29	80-95*	fiberglass or Kevlar
Nimbus Kiska (tandem)	18'	28	78-92*	fiberglass or Kevlar
Nimbus Lootas Series	18'6"	23	48-56*	fiberglass or Kevlar
Nimbus Njak	16'6"	23¾	45-53*	fiberglass or Kevlar
Nimbus Puffin	16'3"	23½	63	polyethylene
Nimbus Seafarer	16'9"	24	48-56*	fiberglass or Kevlar
Nimbus Skana (tandem)	21'7"	30	90-105*	fiberglass or Kevlar
Nimbus Solander Plus	16'2"	23	45-53*	fiberglass or Kevlar
Nimbus Sprint	17'6"	22	45-54*	fiberglass or Kevlar
Nimbus Telkwa Series	18'3"	23¾	52-59*	fiberglass or Kevlar
Seaward (1989)				
Ascente	18'2"	22½	46-56*	fiberglass or Kevlar
Cobra	16'	23	43-53*	fiberglass or Kevlar
Navigator	17'	24½	45-55*	fiberglass or Kevlar
Passat K-2 (tandem)	22'	26	80-95*	fiberglass or Kevlar
Quest	19'	22½	48-58*	fiberglass or Kevlar
Southwind K-2 (tandem)	21'	30½	46-56*	fiberglass or Kevlar
Tyee	17'	24½	45-55*	fiberglass or Kevlar
Vision	17'	24	48-55*	fiberglass or Kevlar
Seda (1969)				
Glider	19'	22	43-56*	fiberglass or Kevlar
Gypsy	15'	24	36-50*	fiberglass, Kevlar, or polyethylene
Impulse	18'	21	41-55*	fiberglass or Kevlar
Swift	17'	24	50	fiberglass
Tango	21'	29	76-95*	fiberglass or polyethylene
Viking	16'6"	25	38-52*	fiberglass or polyethylene
Southern Exposure (1985)				
Naiad	17'3"	20½	52	fiberglass
Reiver	17'2"	20½	52	fiberglass

Keel	Bottom	Sides	Price (dollars)
straight with rise at ends	shallow arch V	flared	550
straight with rise at ends	rounded V	flared	1100
straight with rise at ends	shallow V	flared	1050
straight with rise at ends	shallow V	flared	1200-2900*
straight with rise at ends	flat	flared	800
straight with rise at ends	shallow V	flared	450
straight with rise at ends	shallow V	flared	1200
straight	shallow V	flared	950-1250*
straight	shallow arch	flared	950-1250*
straight with rise at ends	flat	tumblehome	1350-1700*
straight with rise at ends	flat	flared	1350
straight with rise at ends	flat	flared	1100
straight with rise at ends	flat	flared	900
straight with rise at ends	shallow V	flared	2150
straight with rise at ends	shallow V	flared	1750
straight with rise at ends	rounded V	flared	2200-2600*
straight with rise at ends	rounded V	flared	2150-2500*
straight with rise at ends	rounded V	flared	3000-3500*
straight with rise at ends	rounded V	flared	3000-3500*
straight with rise at ends	rounded V	flared	3000-3500*
moderately rockered	rounded V	flared	2200-2600*
straight with rise at ends	rounded V	flared	2150-2500*
straight with rise at ends	rounded V	flared	2200
straight with rise at ends	rounded V	flared	2150-2500*
straight with rise at ends	rounded V	flared	3250-3800*
straight with rise at ends	rounded V	flared	2150-2500*
straight with rise at ends	rounded V	flared	2150-2500*
straight with rise at ends	rounded V	flared	2250-2600*
straight with rise at ends	shallow V	straight	2250-2800*
straight with rise at ends	shallow V	straight	2250-2800*
straight with rise at ends	shallow V	straight	2250-2800*
straight with rise at ends	shallow V	straight	2850-3450*
straight with rise at ends	shallow V	straight	2350-2850*
straight with rise at ends	shallow V	straight	3000-3600*
straight with rise at ends	shallow V	straight	2250-2800*
moderate rocker	rounded V	straight	2250-2600*
straight with rise at ends	shallow V	flared	1250-1800*
straight with rise at ends	shallow V	tumblehome	850-1800*
straight with rise at ends	shallow V	flared	1250-1800*
straight with rise at ends	shallow V	flared	1250
straight with rise at ends	shallow V	flared	1900-2600*
straight with rise at ends	shallow V	flared	1250-1800*
straight with rise at ends	shallow V	flared	1750-2500*
straight with rise at ends	shallow V	flared	1750-2500*

Manufacturer/model	Length (feet)	Width (inches)	Weight (pounds)	Material
Superior (1990)				
Arctic Hawk Series	18', 18'10"	22	42-44*	wood/fiberglass
Hawk	19'2"	21	44	wood/fiberglass
Northern Hawk	19'	23½	46	wood/fiberglass
Sea Hawk	17'4"	21¾	40	wood/fiberglass
Sparrow Hawk	16'6"	21½	37	wood/fiberglass
Swift (1994)				
Caspian Sea	15'3"	24	34	proprietary lay-up
North Sea	16'9"	23	36	proprietary lay-up
The Upstream Edge (1984)				
Sea Lion Series	17', 17'10"	22½, 23	45-58*	fiberglass or Kevlar
Trent (1979)				
Sea Hawk	16'6"	27	42	wood
Tsunami (1986)				
X-15 Scramjet	14'	23	50	Kevlar
Valley Canoe Products (VCP) (1970)				
Aleut Sea II (tandem)	22'	26	80-90*	fiberglass or Kevlar
Anas Acuta	17'2"	20	40-50*	fiberglass or Kevlar
Aquila H	18'3"	22½	48-58*	fiberglass or Kevlar
Greenlander	17'8"	21	40-50*	fiberglass or Kevlar
Nordkapp Series	17'10"	21	45-58*	fiberglass or Kevlar
Pintail Series	17'2"	22	40-50*	fiberglass or Kevlar
Romany Series	16', 17'6"	21½	52-56*	fiberglass or Kevlar
Skerray Series	17', 17'8"	23, 24	56-60*	fiberglass or Kevlar
Vermont Canoe Products (1989)				
Spirit	17'2"	25	53	fiberglass
Walden (1992)				
Vision Series	12'6"	25	40-42*	polyethylene
Vista Series	12'6"	24	41-43*	polyethylene
West Side (1977)				
Baby Otter (children)	9'8"	22	19	fiberglass
Delta	13'10"	24	28	Kevlar
Extra Fast Touring	19'2"	20½	35	Kevlar
Seafarer Series	15'8", 16'8", 17'4", 20'	22, 23, 24, 28	35-75*	fiberglass or Kevlar
Umnak	15'5"	24	35-42*	fiberglass or Kevlar
Wet Willy (1995)				
Javlin	20'	22	56	wood/fiberglass
Quest	15'	23½	49	wood/fiberglass
Spirit	17'	23	53	wood/fiberglass
Wilderness Systems (1986)				
Alto Expedition	16'1"	22	55	polyethylene
Arctic Hawk Series	17'11"	22	42-46*	fiberglass or Kevlar
Echo Series (tandem)	18'	24½	60-70*	fiberglass or Kevlar
Epic	17'	22	59	polyethylene
Piccolo	13'5"	20	59	polyethylene
Poquito	12'	20½	25-30*	fiberglass or Kevlar
Seacret Expedition	14'6"	25½	57	polyethylene
Sealution Series	16'6", 18'	21½-24	45-60*	fiberglass or Kevlar

Keel	Bottom	Sides	Price (dollars)
straight with rise at ends	shallow V	flared	3200-3300*
straight with rise at ends	shallow V	flared	3300
straight with rise at ends	shallow V	flared	3300
straight with rise at ends	shallow V	flared	3200
straight with rise at ends	shallow V	flared	3200
moderate rocker	rounded V	flared	1600
moderate rocker	rounded V	flared	1650
straight	shallow V	flared	2400-2800*
straight with rise at ends	shallow arch	flared	1650
extreme rocker	shallow arch	tumblehome	2500
straight with rise at ends	shallow arch	flared	2150-2650*
straight with rise at ends	shallow arch	flared	1650-2150*
straight with rise at ends	shallow arch	flared	1950-2450*
straight with rise at ends	shallow arch	flared	1850-2350*
straight with rise at ends	shallow arch	flared	2000-2500*
straight with rise at ends	shallow arch	flared	2000-2500*
straight with rise at ends	rounded	flared	1850-2350*
straight with rise at ends	rounded	flared	1950-2450*
straight with rise at ends	shallow arch	straight	1250
straight with rise at ends	rounded V	flared	700-850*
straight with rise at ends	rounded V	flared	600-700*
extreme rocker	rounded V	straight	550
straight with rise at ends	deep V	flared	1250
moderate rocker	rounded V	flared	1800
moderate rocker	shallow arch	flared	1800-2700*
straight with rise at ends	shallow V	flared	1800*
straight with rise at ends	shallow V	flared	2900
moderate rocker	shallow V	straight	2400
moderate rocker	shallow V	straight	2650
straight with rise at ends	shallow V	flared	850
straight with rise at ends	deep V	flared	1750-2250*
straight with rise at ends	rounded V	flared	2350-3300*
straight with rise at ends	shallow V	flared	1150
moderate rocker	rounded V	tumblehome	650
straight with rise at ends	rounded V	tumblehome	950-1500*
moderate rocker	shallow V	tumblehome	800
moderate rocker	shallow V	tumblehome	800*

Manufacturer/model	Length (feet)	Width (inches)	Weight (pounds)	Material
Wilderness Systems Continued				
Sealution II Series	14'6"-17'	22-23½	52-60*	polyethylene
Sea-Two (tandem)	17'3"	30	90	polyethylene
Shenai Series	17'4"	22	45*	fiberglass or Kevlar
Skookumchuck (tandem)	21'	32	80-90*	fiberglass or Kevlar
Sparrow Hawk Series	16'6"	21½	38-42*	fiberglass or Kevlar
Tchaika Series	14'	21¾	40-42*	fiberglass or Kevlar
Woodstrip Watercraft (1987)				
Auk Series	15'3", 17'	21-23	40-45*	wood
DD 17	15'9'	22	35	wood
DD 21	15'10'	22½	35	wood
Dovekie Series	14'10", 16'6"	23-26	40-45*	wood
Razorbill Series	15'11", 17'8"	21-23	40-45*	wood
Skimmer	21'1'	26	65	wood

(Year in parentheses is year the company began making boats)
* Depending on model, material, or options
** Also available in a smaller version designed for women

Keel	Bottom	Sides	Price (dollars)
moderate rocker	shallow V	straight	1000-1200*
moderate rocker	shallow V	tumblehome	1450
straight with rise at ends	rounded V	flared	1700-2550*
moderate rocker	rounded V	straight	2850-3500*
straight with rise at ends	deep V	flared	1750-2550*
moderate rocker	rounded V	tumblehome	1250-1950*
straight with rise at ends	shallow V	flared	2300-2600*
straight with rise at ends	deep V	flared	1850
straight with rise at ends	round V	flared	1850
straight with rise at ends	shallow V	flared	2300-2600*
straight with rise at ends	rounded V	flared	2600-2700*
straight with rise at ends	shallow V	flared	3600

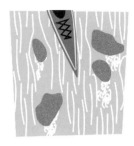

Chapter 7
Whitewater Kayaks

Few endeavors are more exciting to watch—or to participate in—than whitewater kayaking. The river represents the absolute in a current-dominated environment. Strokes are made to take advantage of the current rather than to propel the kayak from put-in to take-out. The key factor here is maneuverability. A boat that tracks down a straight line and resists deviating from its course isn't desirable in this realm.

at the waterline, which reduces the amount of surface the current can grab.

A buoyant boat will be a relatively forgiving boat—tolerant of mistakes and able to bob through some significant stretches of whitewater. Buoyancy, however, is a double-edged sword. Although it is easy to keep afloat, this relatively high-volume kayak will be bounced around in the waves and currents and give the paddler a real workout.

Whitewater Kayak Design

A shorter kayak is more maneuverable and turns more easily but has less straight-line tracking ability than a longer one. Straight-line speed is lost in the process, but top speed is less critical on the river. To gain even more maneuverability for ferrying across the current and turning in and out of eddies, whitewater kayaks typically feature increased rocker at the bow and stern. This upsweep in the keel makes the kayak easier to turn and spin because the boat is shorter

Whitewater Readiness

The best measures for safety and success on the river are preventative: sharpening wilderness skills, staying in good physical condition, keeping equipment in good repair, and researching the territory you plan to cover. Accidents do happen, even to the most experienced paddler, but being prepared just makes sense.

It's always a good idea to start on easy rivers early in the season and gain some experience before moving on to more difficult

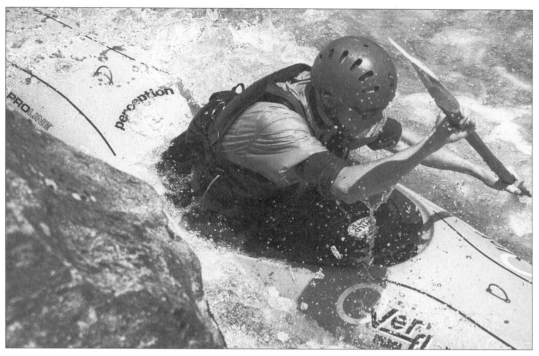

(courtesy Lotus Designs)

water. When running any river you're not familiar with, collect everything you can: guidebooks, maps, magazine articles, and reports from other boaters.

Reading Whitewater

The art of looking at a stretch of whitewater to determine where the hazards lie is a talent developed only by experience. Personal instruction can help, but no book or video can do justice to the nuances of the art.

The whitewater kayaker is constantly looking downstream to determine the hydraulics of the river, and specifically, where water flows over a rock and then back on itself, a situation known as a reversal or hole. Small holes present little trouble. But there are holes that can stop a boat—appro-

priately called stoppers. Larger ones yet—called keepers—can hold and recirculate a boat for what seems like indefinitely.

Instructional Videos

Excellent videos for learning the techniques of whitewater paddling are *The Kayaker's Edge,* by Kent Ford, and *Essential Boat Control,* by Tom Decuir.

Recommended videos for learning rescue techniques are *River Rescue* and *Heads Up: River Rescue for River Runners.* (See Chapter 15 for information on kayak safety and rescue.)

All of these videos can be purchased from Four Corners River Sports, P.O. Box 379, Durango, CO 81302; (800) 426–7637.

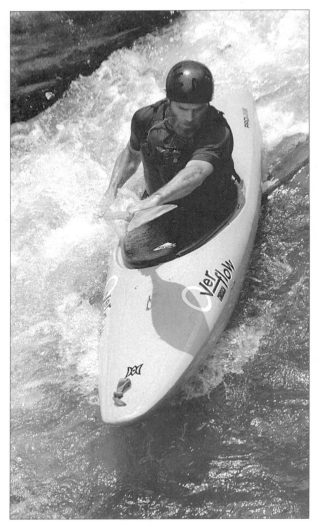

(courtesy Lotus Designs)

International Scale of Whitewater Difficulty

Class I—Easy. This is the most minor of rapids, with very small waves and easily avoided obstacles.

Class II—Novice. Again, these are easy rapids, but there is some maneuvering required.

Class III—Intermediate. Things are starting to advance. Waves are more numerous, and some may be quite high. Rocks arise, and so there is the need for good maneuvering skills. It may even be necessary to scout the rapids.

Class IV—Advanced. These are long, powerful rapids with many irregularities that require skill to read. Precise maneuvering is required, as is scouting of the rapids. Most importantly, there is a risk of capsizing the boat. This level is for very skilled kayakers with a lot of experience.

Class V—Expert. Here there is a risk of serious injury, even to well-qualified paddlers. The currents are so complicated and convoluted that they seem indistinguishable. Scouting is mandatory, though it may be difficult. Rescue stations must be established downstream due to the high likelihood of error.

Class VI—Extreme. Most boaters consider this level to be unrunnable; it is that dangerous.

To determine whether a hole is hazardous or not, a kayaker must look for signs, which is difficult to do because of the kayaker's close proximity to the surface of the water. Irregular waves are one indicator. A calm spot in the midst of turbulence is another. Even the sound of the rapid can make the boater aware there is a problem. Ultimately, experience is the only reliable guide to reading whitewater.

Safety Gear for Whitewater Kayaking

The following are considered essential safety items for whitewater boaters. (See Chapter 15 for a complete discussion.)
- Personal flotation device.

- Helmets.
- A throw-rope. For rescue of other boaters.
- Rescue lines. For boat rescue.
- First-aid kit.
- Repair kit.
- River knives. Helpful to avoid entanglement with ropes, as well as other uses.
- Sponge or bilge pump.
- Whistle. To communicate with other boaters at a distance.
- Gloves. To avoid blisters.

The Builders

Among the manufacturers of whitewater kayaks are Phoenix Poke Boats and Prijon, and some of their boats are discussed here. You'll find statistical details on whitewater kayaks made by these and other manufacturers in the fact grids that follow this section.

Phoenix Poke Boats

Phoenix Poke Boats, of Berea, Kentucky, has been building boats since 1973. Its boats are made of fiberglass or Kevlar.

The 13-foot, 2-inch Cascade is a classic whitewater design with a V bow and stern that contributes to speed and tracking. Rounded sides permit body balance turns. Large volume provides room for big paddlers and gear, and it adds buoyancy as well. The Cascade is a good choice for beginners. The boat weighs 27 pounds in fiberglass, 23 pounds in Kevlar. Price: $950 (fiberglass); $1250 (Kevlar).

At 13 feet, 9 inches long and 24½ inches wide, the Appalachian is a big Cascade, best for paddlers over 165 pounds. The boat weighs 34 pounds in fiberglass or 28

Where To Go?

Two books that can help you decide where you would like to kayak are *The Whitewater Sourcebook: A Directory of Information on American Whitewater Rivers,* by Richard Penny (Birmingham, Alabama: Menasha Ridge Press, 1991) and *Western Whitewater: From the Rockies to the Pacific,* by Jim Cassady, Bill Cross, and Fryar Calhoun (Berkeley: North Fork Press, 1994).

Here's a "wish list" of several favored rivers for whitewater kayakers:

East
Youghiogheny (Maryland, Pennsylvania)
Cheat (West Virginia)
New (West Virginia)
Gauley (West Virginia)
Chattooga (Georgia, South Carolina)
Penobscot (Maine)

West
American (California)
Stanislaus (California)
Tuolumne (California)
Kern (California)
Salmon (Idaho)
Rogue (Oregon)
Snake (Wyoming, Idaho/Oregon)
Colorado (Arizona)
Green (Utah)

pounds in Kevlar. Price: $950 (fiberglass); $1250 (Kevlar).

The Seewun, at 13 feet, 2 inches, is a whitewater touring boat that runs rivers more readily than a canoe. For advanced and expert kayakers, it offers an opportunity to get a thrill out of easier rivers. The Seewun's high volume promotes stability, while high rocker makes it easy to turn. The

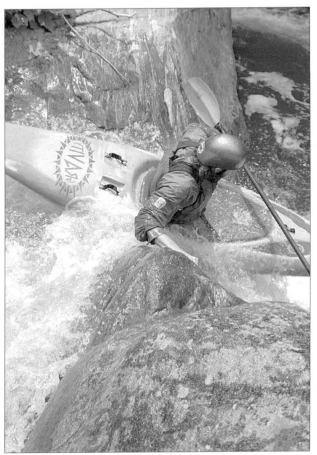

(courtesy Lotus Designs)

weight is 28 pounds in fiberglass or 23 pounds in Kevlar. Price: $950 (fiberglass); $1250 (Kevlar).

Prijon

Prijon is a German manufacturer whose boats are distributed in the United States by Wildwasser Sports in Boulder, Colorado. All of its whitewater boats are made of polyethylene.

The Cyclone is a versatile whitewater boat designed not only for playing in holes and surfing waves, but to provide performance between play spots. A slightly upturned bow helps prevent diving while surfing. A sleek design lets the boat pierce waves and haystacks while still providing sufficient volume to reliably surface. Prijon recommends the Cyclone, which is 10 feet, 6 inches long and weighs 41 pounds, for women, juniors, and smaller paddlers. Price: $850.

The Canyon is offered as a whitewater boat suitable for both experts and beginners. It is designed to provide stability and responsiveness that help the expert in demanding whitewater and that also assist the beginner because the boat is not overly sensitive. The Canyon—11 feet long and weighing 44 pounds—has sufficient volume to handle a larger paddler and gear for extended excursions. Price: about $850.

The Tornado is designed to appeal to large paddlers and to kayakers who need an

Olympic Kayak Coach

The most famous coach of Olympic kayakers is Bill Endicott, who has written a number of books on the subject:

The River Masters: A History of the World Championships of Whitewater Canoeing (Washington, D.C.: Endicott)

The Ultimate Run: Canoe Slalom at the Highest Levels (Baltimore: Reese Press, 1983)

The Danger Zone: Downriver Canoeing at the Highest Levels (Baltimore: Reese Press, 1985)

Also of interest to Olympic watchers is *Canoeing: An Olympic Sport*, by Andras "Andy" Toro (San Francisco: Olympian Graphics, 1986)

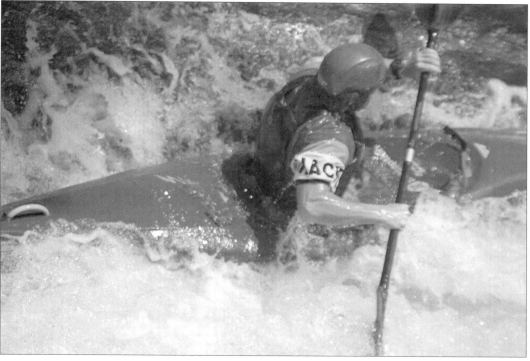

(courtesy Lotus Designs)

expedition-grade boat for self-supported whitewater trips. A pronounced rocker and generous bow volume assist in resurfacing quickly after big drops, and a blunt profile helps prevent vertical pinning. The Tornado, at 11 feet, 5 inches in length, weighs 46 pounds. Price: about $850.

The expedition-proven Yukon Tour pro-vides a trihedral hull cross-section credited with improving stability, speed, and maneuverability. The design, with a low profile, is aimed at good tracking in windy situations. Large storage capacity in both bow and stem of the 44-pound boat is easily accessed; the seat back is detachable. The Yukon is 14 feet, 5 inches long. Cost: about $850.

Whitewater Kayaks

The following grids present details on the lineup of whitewater kayaks offered by selected manufacturers. See the end of this chapter for the addresses and phone numbers of these and other manufacturers. For information on paddles, see Chapter 3. For information on spray skirts, life jackets, and other accessories, see Chapter 14.

Manufacturer/model	Length (feet)	Width (inches)	Weight (pounds)	Material
Baldwin (1966)				
Downriver K-1 Series	13'2"	24	21-35*	fiberglass or Kevlar
Slalom K-1 Series	13'2"	24	20-32*	fiberglass or Kevlar
Dagger (1988)				
Predator Series	13'2"	24	20	Kevlar
Profile	13'2"	24	20	Kevlar
Englehart (1988)				
Epidart	13'2"	24	23	proprietary lay-up
Epilight	13'2"	24	23	proprietary lay-up
Kiwi (1988)				
Lobo	9'2"	29	37	polyethylene
Massive (1994)				
Skimmer	11'3"	24	28-34*	fiberglass, Kevlar, or proprietary lay-up
Millbrook (1995)				
Dinger	13'2"	24	20*	fiberglass or Kevlar
Phoenix Poke Boats (1973)				
Appalachian	13'9"	24½	28-34*	proprietary lay-up or Kevlar
Cascade	13'2"	24	23-27*	proprietary lay-up or Kevlar
Seewun	13'2"	27½	23-28*	proprietary lay-up or Kevlar
Prijon (1985)				
Slalom	12'3"	24	42	polyethylene
Tornado	11'5"	25	46	polyethylene
Seda (1969)				
Climax	13'2"	24	25-32*	fiberglass or Kevlar
Crest	11'6"	24	34	polyethylene
The Upstream Edge (1984)				
Bravo	13'2"	24	18-28*	fiberglass or Kevlar
Mystery Series	13'2"	24	19-28*	fiberglass or Kevlar
Nomad Extra	13'2"	24	18-24*	fiberglass or Kevlar
Prijon Sanna	13'2"	24	18-28*	fiberglass or Kevlar
Prijon Treska	13'2"	24	18-24*	fiberglass or Kevlar
Reflex Series	13'2"	24	18-24*	fiberglass or Kevlar
Super Glide	13'2"	24	18-28*	fiberglass or Kevlar
Vermont Canoe Products (1989)				
Osprey	13'4"	23	35	fiberglass
West Side (1977)				
Bala Racer	13'2"	24	19	Kevlar

(Year in parentheses is year the company began making boats)
* Depending on model, material, or options

Keel	Bottom	Sides	Price (dollars)
straight ends	shallow V	tumblehome	750-1250*
extreme rocker	shallow V	tumblehome	700-1100*
extreme rocker	flat	straight	1600
extreme rocker	flat	straight	1600
extreme rocker	shallow arch	flared	1950
extreme rocker	shallow arch	flared	1950
straight with rise at ends	shallow V	straight	450
extreme rocker	shallow arch	flared	950-1300*
extreme rocker	flat	straight	750-1000*
straight with rise at ends	shallow arch	tumblehome	950-1250*
moderate rocker	shallow arch	tumblehome	950-1250*
moderate rocker	shallow arch	tumblehome	950-1250*
moderate rocker	flat	straight	750
extreme rocker	shallow arch	tumblehome	860
moderate rocker	rounded V	tumblehome	800-1100*
extreme rocker	shallow arch	straight	600
extreme rocker	flat	flared	1150-1600*
extreme rocker	flat	flared	1150-1600*
extreme rocker	flat	flared	1150-1600*
extreme rocker	flat	flared	1150-1600*
extreme rocker	flat	flared	1150-1600*
extreme rocker	flat	flared	1150-1600*
extreme rocker	flat	flared	1150-1600*
extreme rocker	shallow arch	tumblehome	650
extreme rocker	rounded V	straight	1250

Whitewater Kayak Manufacturers

Aquaterra
(See Perception)

Baldwin Boat Company
RR 2, Box 268
Orrington, ME 04474
(207) 825–4439

Competition Kayak
P.O. Box 31064
Albuquerque, NM 87190
(505) 888–5800
Fax (505) 888–7912

Dagger Canoe Company
P.O. Box 1500
Harriman, TN 37748
(423) 882–0404
Fax (423) 882–8153

Englehart Products Inc. (EPI)
P.O. Box 377
Newbury, OH 44065
(216) 564–5565
Fax (216) 564–5515

Euro Kayaks/TG Canoe Livery
P.O. Box 177
Martindale, TX 78655
(512) 353–3946
Fax (512) 353–3947

Great Canadian Canoe Company
64 Worcester Providence Turnpike
Sutton, MA 01590
(508) 865–0010
Fax (508) 865–5220

Hydra Kayaks
5061 South National Drive
Knoxville, TN 37914

Guidebooks

Following is a selected list of useful state guidebooks:

Alaska River Guide: Canoeing, Kayaking, and Rafting in the Last Frontier, by Karen Jettmar (Seattle: Alaska Northwest Books, 1993)

Fast and Cold: A Guide to Alaska Whitewater, by Andrew Embick (Skyhouse: 1994)

Idaho—The Whitewater State: A Guidebook, by Grant Amaral (Boise, Idaho: Watershed Books, 1989)

Canoe and Kayak Routes of Northwest Oregon, by Philip N. Jones (Seattle: The Mountaineers, 1997)

California Whitewater: A Guide to the Rivers (third edition), by Jim Cassady and Fryar Calhoun (Berkeley: North Fork Press, 1997)

Appalachian Whitewater (two volumes), by Bob Schlinger (Birmingham, Alabama: Menasha Ridge Press, 1994)

Carolina Whitewater, by Bob Benner and David Benner (Menasha Ridge Press, 1997)

Wildwater West Virginia (third edition), by Paul Davidson (Menasha Ridge Press, 1997)

Among the catalog companies that stock guidebooks of interest to river runners are Adventurous Traveler Bookstore, P.O. Box 64769, Burlington, VT 05406 (800–282–3963) and GORP, P.O. Box 3016, Everett, WA 98203 (888–994–4677).

(800) 537–8888
Fax (305) 836–1296

Impex International
(See Pyranha)

Kiwi Kayak Company
2454 Vista Del Monte
Concord, CA 94520
(510) 692–2041
Fax (510) 692–2042

Massive
3976 Highway 17
Kinburn, Ontario K0A 2H0
(613) 832–1416
Fax (613) 832–0350

Necky Kayaks
1100 Riverside Road
Abbotsford, British Columbia
V2S 7P1
(604) 850–1206
Fax (604) 850–3197

Northwest Kayaks
15145 NE 90th Street
Redmond, WA 98052
(425) 869–1107
Fax (425) 869–9014

Perception, Inc.
P.O. Box 8002
Easley, SC 29641
(803) 859–7518
Fax (803) 855–5995

Phoenix Poke Boats
P.O. Box 109
207 N. Broadway
Berea, KY 40403-0109

Kayaking on the Edge

Looking for exciting reading on white-water kayaking adventure? Try the books *First Descents: In Search of Wild Rivers,* edited by Cameron O'Connor and John Lazenby (Birmingham, Alabama: Menasha Ridge Press, 1989), and *Class V Chronicles,* edited by Jeff Bennett (Portland, Oregon: Swiftwater Publishing, 1992). It's guaranteed that you won't be able to put these stories down.

The Amazon has always appealed to adventurers, and kayakers are no different. A couple of good boating reads about paddling this river are *Running the Amazon,* by Joe Kane (New York: Vintage Books, 1990) and *Demon River Apurimac: The First Navigation of Upper Amazon Canyons,* by Calvin Giddings (Salt Lake City: University of Utah Press, 1996). These books describe the heights of a challenging kayak adventure.

(606) 986–2336
Fax (606) 986–3277

Prijon/Wildwasser Sport USA
P.O. Box 4617
Boulder, CO 80306
(303) 444–2336
Fax (303) 444–2375

Pyranha/Impex International
1107 Station Road
Bellport, NY 11713
(516) 286–1988
Fax (516) 286–1952

Good Reads: Whitewater Kayaking

Kayaking: Whitewater and Touring Basics, by Steven M. Krauzer (New York: W. W. Norton, 1995)

Wildwater: The Sierra Club Guide to Kayaking and Whitewater Boating, by Lito Tejada-Flores (San Francisco: Sierra Club Books, 1978)

Whitewater Handbook (third edition), by Bruce Lessels (Boston: Appalachian Mountain Club Books, 1994)

The Kayaking Book, by Jay Evans and Eric Evans (New York: NAL/Dutton, 1993)

Performance Kayaking, by Stephen U'Ren (Mechanicsburg, Pennsylvania: Stackpole Books, 1996)

White Water Kayaking, by Ray Rowe (Mechanicsburg, Pennsylvania: Stackpole Books, 1989)

Savage Designs
2000 Riverside Drive
Asheville, NC 28804
(704) 251–9875
Fax (704) 285–0607

Seda Products
926 Coolidge Avenue
National City, CA 91950
(619) 336–2444
Fax (619) 336–2405

The Upstream Edge (Rockwood Outfitters)
699 Speedvale Avenue West
Guelph, Ontario N1K 1E6
(519) 824–1415
Fax (519) 824–8750

Tsunami
13732 Bear Mountain Road
Redding, CA 96003
(916) 275–4313
Fax (916) 275–3090

Vermont Canoe Products
R.R. 1, Box 353A
Newport, VT 05855
(800) 454–2307
Fax (802) 754–2307

Wave Sport
P.O. Box 5207
Steamboat Springs, CO 80477
(970) 736–0080
Fax (970) 736–0078

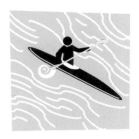

Chapter 8
Whitewater Playboats

Kayaking has always had its share of plea-surable moments of playing in the waves and currents, but the emphasis is usually on moving from point A to point B. Many whitewater boaters prefer instead to focus on playing in one area. A whitewater play-boat is made specifically for the currents of a river, as is its close relative, the squirt boat, which can maneuver through under-water currents.

Playboat Design

Playboats are specially designed kayaks for performing stunts in the holes, waves, and pour-overs of a whitewater river. These tricks include spinning in holes, doing enders (where the kayak is suddenly propelled out of the water like a rocket), and wave surfing. Whitewater playboats are usually less than 12 feet long and have a pronounced rocker, because these features allow the kayak to turn quickly. Playboaters compete against one another in contests called white-water rodeos, which are held around the country and attract the best in the sport.

Squirt boats are a bit smaller, a bit rounder, and even more feisty and chal-lenging. See the end of this chapter for a brief look at squirt boating and some se-lected models.

Safety Gear for Playboating

The following are considered essential safety items for playboaters (see Chapter 15 for a complete discussion).

- Personal flotation device
- Helmet
- A throw-rope
- Rescue line
- First-aid kit
- Repair kit
- River knife
- Sponge or bilge pump
- Whistle
- Gloves

The Builders

Among the manufacturers of whitewater playboats are Dagger and Euro, and some of their boats are discussed here. You'll find statistical details on whitewater playboats made by these and other manufacturers in the fact grids that follow this section.

Dagger

Dagger Canoe Company, of Harriman, Tennessee, has been building boats since 1988. It is one of the largest kayak manufacturers in the country and its wide array

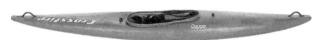

Dagger Canoe Co.'s Crossfire

of playboats are made of polyethylene.

The Vertigo is Dagger's latest entry in the market for rodeo playboats. Designed by Mark Lyle and Steve Scarborough, the Vertigo's flat hull, roto-molded seat, and hard chines make for a boat that spins readily. Its volume is distributed in a way that aids hard-to-make retentive moves. The length is only 7 feet, 11 inches, and weight is 32 pounds. Price: $900.

The 9-foot-long RPM is Dagger's best seller, touted for an agility in linking cartwheels, shredding waves, or running a river. Price: $900.

The Gradient is a high-performance

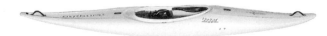

Dagger Canoe Co.'s Outburst

creek boat with features that include a recessed deck area for a throw rope, smooth chines, and radical rocker for tight moves. The Gradient combines short length (8 feet, 8 inches), high volume, and fast acceleration. Price: $900.

Dagger recommends its 9-foot, 5-inch Freefall LT for hard-core creek kayakers and beginning boaters alike. Good maneuverability, stability, and volume are cited as factors in making the Freefall LT suitable for the expert on tight, technical runs and also for beginning or intermediate kayakers looking for steep drops. The LT can handle enough gear for overnight and self-contained trips. Price: about $900.

Designed as an all-purpose, high-performance kayak for smaller folks, the Blast works for surfing, hole playing, and general river running. The Blast's seat and thigh braces are specially formed to fit smaller body types, and it's a good first boat for

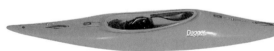

Dagger Canoe Co.'s RPM

kids. It can also be used by larger paddlers as a rodeo boat. The Blast is 9 feet, 5 inches long and weighs 30 pounds. Price: $800.

The 11-foot Crossfire offers soft chines and high bow buoyancy for stability and predictability, even when punching through big holes and standing waves. It's offered as a choice for big-water paddlers who want a forgiving design and substantial storage capacity. Price: $900.

The Outburst is termed a hybrid, promising river-running stability with play-

Playboat Lingo

Playboaters have a language of their own. If you spend any time in these boating circles, you'll no doubt hear terms like:

Airtime: Any pop-up, or pirouette, that is vertical.

Boof: A safety move off of a drop, landing nearly flat behind a rock in calm water.

Ender (or endo, or pop-up): Using a hydraulic to stand your boat up vertically.

McTwist: Angled spin, using water pressure on your deck to spin you around.

Retendo (retentive ender): An ender that lands you back in the hole.

Surfing: Riding a river hydraulic like an ocean wave—except that on a river, you and the wave are stationary.

Three-sixty: A flat spin—a full 360 degrees around—with your deck out of the water.

Whippet: A vertical 180-degree move, side to side, like a cartwheel.

boat spirit. A low-volume bow and stern are designed for play moves, while a long waterline and midsection contribute to speed and buoyancy for running the whitewater. The Outburst measures 10 feet, 10 inches. Price: $900.

Euro

Euro-Kayaks is a German manufacturer whose products are distributed in the United States from Martindale, Texas. Its playboats are made of polyethylene.

The Rapid Fire, created by designer Klaus Lettmann, is Euro Kayak's latest model. The pronounced rocker and short waterline on this 10-foot playboat promote maneuverability for surfing and wave-riding. Lower volume at the front and rear decks aids performance, while increased volume around the keyhole-cockpit area is aimed at comfort and security for the paddler. Price: $900.

Euro-Kayaks' other new design, the 10-foot, 4-inch Conquest, was originally designed by Trevor Snook for female and smaller paddlers. However, many heavier paddlers use it for negotiating reversals and

standing waves. Its short length and fairly pronounced rocker give it turning abilities that make it a good choice for kayakers progressing from flat to moving water. Price: $900.

The 11-foot Olymp, designed by Klaus Lettmann, is described as a safe and predictable kayak that suits the larger paddler in heavy whitewater. Well-defined rocker and rails make it good for running waterfalls and rapids. The Olymp weighs 44 pounds. Price: $900.

Playboat Manufacturers

Competition Kayak
    P.O. Box 31064
    Albuquerque, NM 87190
    (505) 888–5800
    Fax (505) 888–7912

Dagger Canoe Company
    P.O. Box 1500
    Harriman, TN 37748
    (423) 882–0404
    Fax (423) 882–8153

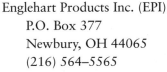

Englehart Products Inc. (EPI)
P.O. Box 377
Newbury, OH 44065
(216) 564–5565
Fax (216) 564–5515

Eskimo Kayaks
3721 Shallow Brook
Bloomfield Hills, MI 48302
(248) 644–6909
Fax (248) 644–4960

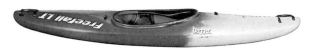

Dagger Canoe Co.'s Freefall

Euro-Kayaks/TG Canoe Livery
P.O. Box 177
Martindale, TX 78655
(512) 353–3946
Fax (512) 353–3947

Great Canadian Canoe Company
64 Worcester Providence Turnpike
Sutton, MA 01590
(508) 865–0010
Fax (508) 865–5220

Hydra Kayaks
5061 South National Drive
Knoxville, TN 37914
(800) 537–8888
Fax (305) 836–1296

Massive
3976 Highway 17
Kinburn, Ontario K0A 2H0
(613) 832–1416
Fax (613) 832–0350

Necky Kayaks
1100 Riverside Road
Abbotsford, British Columbia
V2S 7P1
(604) 850–1206
Fax (604) 850–3197

Northwest Kayaks
15145 NE 90th Street
Redmond, WA 98052
(425) 869–1107
Fax (425) 869–9014

Perception, Inc.
P.O. Box 8002
Easley, SC 29641
(803) 859–7518
Fax (803) 855–5995

Phoenix Poke Boats
P.O. Box 109
207 North Broadway
Berea, KY 40403-0109
(606) 986–2336
Fax (606) 986–3277

Prijon/Wildwasser Sport USA
P.O. Box 4617
Boulder, CO 80306
(303) 444–2336
Fax (303) 444–2375

Good Read: Playboating

Catch Every Eddy, Surf Every Wave: A Contemporary Guide to Whitewater Playboating, by Thomas S. Foster (Outdoor Centre of New England, 1995)

Pyranha/Impex International
1107 Station Road
Bellport, NY 11713
(516) 286–1988
Fax (516) 286–1952

Savage Designs
2000 Riverside Drive
Asheville, NC 28804
(704) 251–9875
Fax (704) 285–0607

Seda Products
926 Coolidge Avenue
National City, CA 91950
(619) 336–2444
Fax (619) 336–2405

The Upstream Edge (Rockwood Outfitters)
699 Speedvale Avenue West
Guelph, Ontario N1K 1E6
(519) 824–1415
Fax (519) 824–8750

Tsunami
13732 Bear Mountain Road
Redding, CA 96003
(916) 275–4313
Fax (916) 275–3090

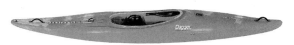

Dagger Canoe Co.'s Animas

Wave Sport
P.O. Box 5207
Steamboat Springs, CO 80477
(970) 736–0080
Fax (970) 736–0078

West Side Boat Shop
7661 Tanawanda Creek Road
Lockport, NY 14094
(716) 434–5755

Playboat Videos

Veteran kayaker Kent Ford has produced a how-to video for playboaters, *Solo Playboating*. Also of interest is the instructional video *Freestylin' Retendo!: The Art of Precision Playpaddling*.

The video *Take the Wild Ride* is freestyle kayaking with the world's best playboaters at the Whitewater Rodeo World Championships on Tennessee's renowned Ocoee River (the site of the 1996 Summer Olympics whitewater course).

These videos are available from Four Corners River Sports, P.O. Box 379, Durango, CO 81302; (800) 426–7637.

Whitewater Playboats

The following grids present details on the lineup of whitewater playboats offered by selected manufacturers. See above for the addresses and phone numbers of these and other manufacturers. For information on paddles, see Chapter 3. For information on spray skirts, life jackets, and other accessories, see Chapter 14.

Manufacturer/model	Length (feet)	Width (inches)	Weight (pounds)	Material
Competition (1996)				
Cosmic 2	10'5"	24½	42	polyethylene
69	18'10"	23½	36	polyethylene
Dagger (1988)				
Animas Series	9'6", 10'5"	23½, 24½	39-40*	polyethylene
Blast	9'5"	22½	30	polyethylene
Crossfire	11'	23¾	38	polyethylene
Freefall LT	9'5"	24	40	polyethylene
Gradient	8'8"	24½	43	polyethylene
Outburst	10'10"	24	40	polyethylene
RPM	9'	24½	37	polyethylene
Vertigo	7'11"	24½	32	polyethylene
Englehart (1988)				
Epiblast	12'	24	26	proprietary lay-up
Epicycloid	11'	24	25	proprietary lay-up
Epimean (designed for women)	10'8"	22½	35	polyethylene
Epitike (designed for children)	9'2"	18½	25	polyethylene
Eskimo (1985)				
Creek/Playboat	9'10"	24	45	polyethylene
Diablo	9'10"	25	42	polyethylene
Kendo	8'6"	25	35	polyethylene
Topolino Series (including tandem)	7'2", 12'1"	24, 26	35, 65*	polyethylene
Euro (1986)				
Blitz	8'6"	24	38	polyethylene
Conquest	10'4"	23	39	polyethylene
Cyphur	10'6"	24	42	polyethylene
Mosquito	10'6"	24	39	polyethylene
Olymp	11'	24½	44	polyethylene
Pinball	6'8"	24	33	polyethylene
Rapid Fire	10'	23½	38	polyethylene
Sunburst Jr.	9'1"	22	30	polyethylene
Thunderbird	8'8"	24	37	polyethylene
Great Canadian (1972)				
R-7	12'	24½	33	polyethylene
Shogun	11'6"	24	35	polyethylene
Hydra (1992)				
Dragonfly II	11'10"	24½	46	polyethylene
Massive (1994)				
Groove K1 Surface	8'1"	26	25-30*	fiberglass, Kevlar, or proprietary lay-up
Necky (1983)				
Jive	8'4"	24	40	polyethylene
Rip	9'2"	23	40	polyethylene
Northwest (1979)				
Photon Series	8'3", 8'7"	23-23¾	26-34*	polyethylene
Perception (1995)				
Arc	9'3"	24½	46	polyethylene
Corsica Series	10'7"-10'10"	23-25	42-46*	polyethylene
Dancer Series	10'4", 11'5"	23-24	35-40*	polyethylene
Fox	11'8"	25	40	polyethylene
Overflow Series	10'-10'1"	23¾-25½	46-48*	polyethylene
Pirouette Series	9'11"-11'2"	23-24	60-69*	polyethylene
Sparc	9'2"	24	40	polyethylene
Whip-It	8'11"	24¼	39	polyethylene
Whiplash	8'11"	24¼	40	polyethylene
3-D	8'2"	24¼	36	polyethylene

Keel	Bottom	Sides	Price (dollars)
extreme rocker	flat	flared	750
extreme rocker	flat	flared	750
extreme rocker	shallow arch	straight	900
extreme rocker	shallow arch	tumblehome	800
extreme rocker	shallow arch	tumblehome	900
extreme rocker	shallow arch	straight	900
extreme rocker	shallow arch	flared	900
extreme rocker	shallow arch	straight	900
extreme rocker	shallow arch	straight	900
extreme rocker	flat	straight	900
extreme rocker	shallow arch	straight	1900
extreme rocker	shallow arch	flared	1800
extreme rocker	shallow arch	straight	600
extreme rocker	shallow arch	straight	500
extreme rocker	flat	flared	950
extreme rocker	flat	flared	950
moderate rocker	flat	tumblehome	950
extreme rocker	shallow arch flat	straight	850-1350*
extreme rocker	shallow arch	flared	900
moderate rocker	shallow arch	tumblehome	900
moderate rocker	shallow arch	tumblehome	900
extreme rocker	shallow arch	flared	900
moderate rocker	shallow arch	tumblehome	900
moderate rocker	flat	flared	900
moderate rocker	shallow arch	flared	900
moderate rocker	shallow V	tumblehome	700
extreme rocker	shallow arch	flared	900
extreme rocker	shallow arch	tumblehome	600
extreme rocker	rounded V	tumblehome	600
moderate rocker	shallow arch	tumblehome	600
extreme rocker	flat	flared	950-1300*
extreme rocker	flat	flared	850
extreme rocker	flat	flared	850
extreme rocker	flat	straight	850-1150*
extreme rocker	flat	straight	900
extreme rocker	flat	flared	750*
extreme rocker	shallow arch	straight	600-750*
straight ends	flat	flared	900
extreme rocker	flat	flared	900
extreme rocker	flat	flared	900
extreme rocker	flat	straight	900
extreme rocker	flat	straight	900
extreme rocker	flat	flared	900
extreme rocker	flat	flared	900

Manufacturer/model	Length (feet)	Width (inches)	Weight (pounds)	Material
Phoenix Poke Boats (1973)				
Micro Slip	12'	24	20-24*	proprietary lay-up or Kevlar
Slipper	13'2"	24	20-24*	proprietary lay-up or Kevlar
Prijon (1962)				
Canyon	11'	24	44	polyethylene
Cyclone	10'6"	24	41	polyethylene
Fly	8'10"	24	37	polyethylene
Hurricane Rodeo	10'2"	25	41	polyethylene
Rockit	9'4"	26	41	polyethylene
Slalom	12'3"	24	42	polyethylene
Pyranha (1974)				
Arco Bat 270	8'10"	23	40	polyethylene
Blade 260	8'8"	23	38	polyethylene
Creek 280	9'	23	40	polyethylene
Migo 230	7'7"	24	38	polyethylene
Migo 240	7'10"	24	40	polyethylene
Mountain 300	10'	24	42	polyethylene
Razor 260	8'8"	23	40	polyethylene
Stunt 300	10'	23	42	polyethylene
Savage Designs (1994)				
Fury	8'6"	24	38	polyethylene
Gravity	10'2"	24	39	polyethylene
Scorpion	10'	24	38	polyethylene
Scream	9'1"	24	39	polyethylene
Seda (1969)				
Cyclone	11'	25	38	polyethylene
Wildcat	9'2"	24	30	polyethylene
The Upstream Edge (1984)				
Pirouette S	10'4"	23	35-40*	fiberglass or Kevlar
Skimmer	11'2"	23	18-28*	fiberglass or Kevlar
Whip-it	8'11"	24	25-30*	fiberglass or Kevlar
Tsunami (1986)				
X-O Crossover	12'6"	24	40	polyethylene
X-7 Mojo	10'7"	23	35	polyethylene
Wave Sports (1987)				
Descente	9'5"	24¾	40	polyethylene
Frankenstein	9'9"	23½	37	polyethylene
Fusion	10'2"	24½	39	polyethylene
Godzilla	8'11"	25½	39	polyethylene
Kinetic	8'8"	23½	37	polyethylene
Micro X	9'11"	24	55	polyethylene
Stubby	7'5"	24½	35	polyethylene
X	8'	24½	37	polyethylene
West Side (1977)				
Otter	13'2"	24	28	Kevlar

(Year in parentheses is year the company began making boats)
*Depending on model, material, or options

Keel	Bottom	Sides	Price (dollars)
extreme rocker	shallow arch	tumblehome	950-1250*
extreme rocker	shallow arch	tumblehome	950-1250*
extreme rocker	shallow arch	tumblehome	850
extreme rocker	shallow arch	tumblehome	850
extreme rocker	shallow arch	flared	850
extreme rocker	flat	flared	900
extreme rocker	flat	flared	850
moderate rocker	flat	straight	725
extreme rocker	shallow arch	flared	900
extreme rocker	flat	straight	900
extreme rocker	shallow arch	flared	900
extreme rocker	shallow arch	flared	900
extreme rocker	shallow arch	flared	900
extreme rocker	shallow arch	flared	900
extreme rocker	flat	straight	900
extreme rocker	shallow arch	flared	900
extreme rocker	flat	tumblehome	850
extreme rocker	flat	flared	850
extreme rocker	shallow arch	straight	850
extreme rocker	shallow arch	flared	850
extreme rocker	shallow arch	straight	700
extreme rocker	flat	tumblehome	700
extreme rocker	shallow arch	tumblehome	1500-1800*
extreme rocker	flat	flared	1150-1600*
extreme rocker	shallow arch	tumblehome	1500-1800*
extreme rocker	shallow arch	tumblehome	1500
extreme rocker	shallow arch	flared	1500
extreme rocker	shallow arch	tumblehome	950
extreme rocker	shallow arch	tumblehome	950
moderate rocker	flat	straight	950
extreme rocker	flat	flared	950
extreme rocker	flat	flared	950
extreme rocker	shallow arch	straight	950
extreme rocker	flat	flared	950
extreme rocker	flat	flared	950
extreme rocker	flat	tumblehome	1250

Squirt Boats

Round out the edges and the ends of a play-boat just a bit, and you have a kayak that's designed to play under the water. It's not a submarine, it's a squirt boat—an acrobat that, in the hands of an experienced paddler, twists and leaps with amazing agility.

The squirt boat, exciting as it is, comes with some serious challenges: It never wants to glide in a straight line, and its space is so confined you have to shoehorn yourself in.

You can read up on these exciting toys in *The Squirt Boat: The Illustrated Boat of Squirt Technique,* by James E. Snyder (Birmingham, Alabama: Menasha Ridge Press, 1987).

If you think playboaters have an unusual language, wait until you hear the murmurings of squirt boaters:

Charc: Charging arc. The angle of attack of a boat's long axis as it encounters currents or other features of the river.

Mystery move: A bow and stern squirt done in close succession so that both ends of the boat sink completely underwater almost simultaneously.

Schnitz: To twirl the paddle around one hand and retrieve it.

Shudder-rudder: To place a rudder stroke directly behind the boat while surfing.

Swirl-o-gram: Any lengthy roll in turbulent waters.

Squirt Boat Manufacturers

Euro-Kayaks/TG Canoe Livery
P.O. Box 177
Martindale, TX 78655
(512) 353–3946
Fax (512) 353–3947

Massive
3976 Highway 17
Kinburn, Ontario K0A 2H0
(613) 832–1416
Fax (613) 832–0350

The Upstream Edge (Rockwood Outfitters)
699 Speedvale Avenue West
Guelph, Ontario N1K 1E6
(519) 824–1415
Fax (519) 824–8750

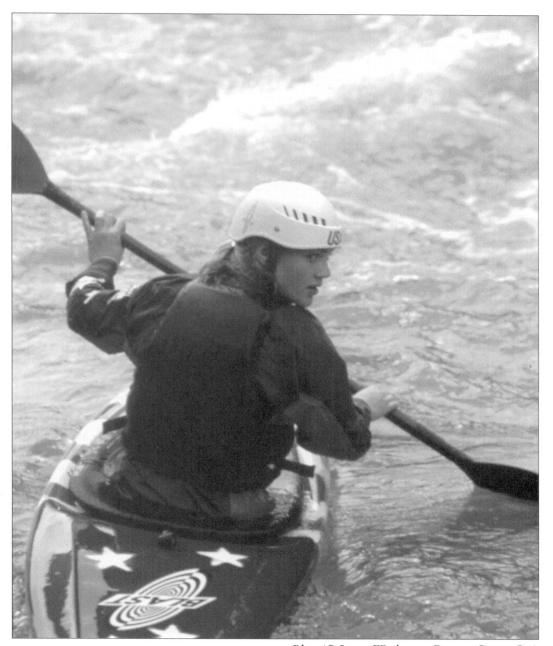

Blast (© Larry Workman, Dagger Canoe Co.)

Squirt Boats

The following grids present details on the lineup of squirt boats offered by Euro Kayaks, Massive, and The Upstream Edge. Addresses for these companies are listed above.

Manufacturer/model	Length (feet)	Width (inches)	Weight (pounds)	Material
Euro (1986)				
Axis	7'11"	24½	32	polyethylene
Enigma	10'	24½	33	polyethylene
Massive (1994)				
Bigfoot	10'	22	22-32*	fiberglass, Kevlar, or proprietary lay-up
Groove K1 Sport	8'1"	26	22-32*	fiberglass, Kevlar, or proprietary lay-up
The Upstream Edge (1984)				
Bigfoot	10'5"	24	25-30*	fiberglass (chopper gun) or Kevlar
Projet	9'6"	23	25-30*	fiberglass (chopper gun) or Kevlar
Shred	10'	23	25-30*	fiberglass (chopper gun) or Kevlar

(Year in parentheses is year the company began making boats)
*Depending on model, material, or options

Keel	Bottom	Sides	Price (dollars)
moderate rocker	shallow arch	tumblehome	800
moderate rocker	shallow arch	tumblehome	775
extreme rocker	shallow arch	flared	950-1300*
extreme rocker	flat	flared	950-1300*
extreme rocker	shallow arch	tumblehome	900-1400*
extreme rocker	shallow arch	tumblehome	900-1400*
extreme rocker	shallow arch	tumblehome	900-1400*

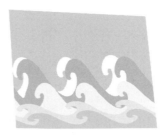

Chapter 9
Surf Kayaks

Kayaks designed specifically for playing in the surf—called wave skis and surf skis—have become just one more extension of the sport of kayaking.

Wave skis are derived from surfboards and are short (usually 6 to 10 feet), feature a blunt nose, and have a fin on the bottom for control. These boats have a very flat hull and a broad, upturned bow shaped like a duck's bill. The cockpit is located a little behind the midpoint and contains the customary bracing of a whitewater kayak. More extreme wave-ski designs are of the sit-on-top variety, which have a shallow seat and two indentations for the feet. This deckless kayak has a hull thick enough to provide sufficient flotation, and the top of the hull is designed so that it holds little water, or is equipped with drain holes.

Surf skis, on the other hand, are long—generally 14 to 18 feet—and resemble a sea kayak in design. They are narrow and have a rudder controlled by the paddler's feet. They are designed to be sat upon rather than in, and have a molded seat and foot well.

Surf kayaks act better than whitewater kayaks in the surf. Whitewater boats knife through the waves rather than riding over them, and their pointed noses cause them to dive into the sand. Compared with a surfboard, a surf kayak offers more comfort—you're sitting rather than standing. And with the kayak's paddle, you are able to maneuver better and travel back out to sea for another ride with greater ease.

The Builders

Among the manufacturers of surf kayaks are Futura and Venturesport, and some of their surf skis are discussed here. You'll find statistical details on surf kayaks (both surf skis and wave skis) from a variety of manufacturers in the fact grids that follow this section.

Futura

Futura, based in National City, California, has been building boats since 1987, and it offers a complete line of surf skis. Its

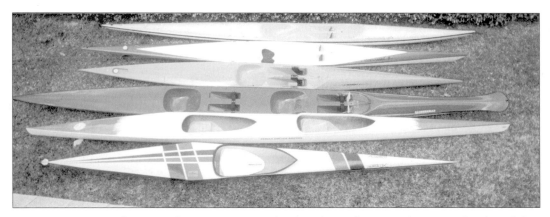

From top to bottom: Elan Crosstrainer, Shearwater, Findeisen, and Hammerhead surf skis, Knysna racing kayak, Excalibur Olympic kayak (courtesy Venturesport, Inc.)

boats are made of a proprietary fiberglass lay-up available in heavy, light, or custom, and all are reinforced in high-stress areas.

The 15-foot Futura has a deep V-shaped bow that cuts through chop and maximizes the waterline length for speed. Options include an 18-by-24-inch enclosed hatch or a regular 12-by-12-inch hatch. Weight is 35 pounds. Price: about $1100.

The 19-foot Futura II was built with the performance paddler in mind—someone seeking a fast boat for racing or touring. Cruising speed is listed at 5 to 6 miles per hour. A small hatch and water bottle holder are available options on this 45-pound surf ski. Price: $1350.

The Blade, at 19 feet, 6 inches long and 17½ inches wide, is a race boat with a shallow seat and deep foot wells to permit an aggressive forward-lean body position for stroking power. Weight is 40 pounds. Price: $1600.

The C-4 is Futura's newest design, with increased rocker and wider beveled seat. This 20-foot boat is available with a skeg rudder to help tracking for both surfing and racing. Price: $1700.

The Futura TS (Tandem Sport) is only slightly longer (20 feet) than many singles on the market, with an efficient hull shape to carry the weight of two people. This 60-pound tandem can also be paddled by just one person. A waterproof hatch is an option. Cost: $1950.

The Futura TR (Tandem Racer), designed to handle two paddlers for racing and fast travel, is 22 feet, 10 inches long and weighs 65 pounds. Price: about $2250.

Venturesport

Venturesport Kayaks & Surf Skis, based in Miami, has been building boats since 1983. Its complete line of surf skis is made of fiberglass or Kevlar.

The Shearwater is Venturesport's fastest surf ski, designed for the speed-minded paddler and serious competitor. Venturesport presents the 20-foot, 6-inch Shearwater as a boat with good speed in both rough ocean and flat-water conditions. It has a deep V hull, sharp entry bow, and narrow hull tapers, helping it slice through the water, while a sloped deck ridge gives the needed volume in the bow to go over waves rather than plowing through them. The shape also helps prevent nosedives when running down-swell. A deep seat-well places the paddler below the waterline for a lower center of gravity, and the foot well is custom-fit to the paddler's leg length. The rudder, always in contact with the water, is designed for minimum drag and turbulence. Weight: 26–33 pounds. Price: $1450–$2050.

The 19-foot Dolphin was designed as a recreational surf ski emphasizing stability, flotation, and seat room. This kayak has conventional lines with high volume and more rocker in the bow. The adjustable foot-well system is offered with an under-stern or over-stern kick-up rudder. The Dolphin EX (expedition option) comes with bow and stern hatches and bulkheads, rear bungie tie-downs, and different lay-up options. Price: $1400.

The Stinger LS promises good handling in extreme surf conditions and when running in following seas, thanks to increased rocker and volume in the bow, along with a built-in bow foil (wave deflector) for vertical and lateral control. This 19-foot boat includes a custom-fit or adjustable foot-well, seat-height option, and under-stern rudder. Fiberglass only. Price: $1450.

The Crosstrainer combines the design of both racing and recreational surf skis. An anatomically designed and formed seat improves comfort for paddling long miles and training. The Crosstrainer has a long, narrow, fish-form rockered V hull with an under-stern rudder. Fiberglass only. Price: about $1500.

Good Reads: Surf Kayaking

The book that concentrates solely on this sport is the new *Surf Kayaking,* by Nigel Foster (The Globe Pequot Press, 1998).

Most of the skills of surf kayaking also can be gleaned from two more general books:

Kayaking: Whitewater and Touring Basics, by Steven M. Krauzer (New York: W. W. Norton, 1995)

The Complete Book of Sea Kayaking, by Derek C. Hutchinson (The Globe Pequot Press, 1995)

Surf Kayak Manufacturers

Euro Kayaks/TG Canoe Livery
    P.O. Box 177
    Martindale, TX 78655
    (512) 353–3946
    Fax (512) 353–3947

Futura Surf Skis
    730 West 19th Street
    National City, CA 91950
    (619) 474–8382
    Fax (619) 474–5167

Island Wave Skis
    2729 South Atlantic Avenue
    Cocoa Beach, FL 32931
    (407) 783–5194
    Fax (407) 783–5194

Karel's Fiberglass Products
    789 Kailua Road
    Kailua HI 96734
    (808) 261–8424
    Fax (808) 261–8424

Mega/Impex International
    1107 Station Road
    Bellport, NY 11713
    (516) 286–1988
    Fax (516) 286–1952

Ocean Kayak
    P.O. Box 5003
    Ferndale, WA 98248
    (800) 852–9257
    Fax (360) 366–2628

Seda Products
    926 Coolidge Avenue
    National City, CA 91950
    (619) 336–2444
    Fax (619) 336–2405

Twogood Kayaks Hawaii
    345 Hahani Street
    Kailua, HI 96734
    (808) 262–5656
    Fax (808) 261–3111
    E-mail: twogood@alohoa.com
    www.alohoa.com\~twogood

Valhalla Surf Ski Products
    4724 Renex Place
    San Diego, CA 92117
    (619) 569–1395
    Fax (619) 569–0295

Venturesport Kayaks & Surf Skis
    P.O. Box 610145
    Miami, FL 33261
    (561) 395–1376

West Side Boat Shop
    7661 Tanawanda Creek Road
    Lockport, NY 14094
    (716) 434–5755

Surf Kayaks

The following grids present details on the lineup of surf kayaks (both surf skis and wave skis) offered by selected manufacturers. See above for the addresses and phone numbers of these and other manufacturers. For information on paddles, see Chapter 3. For information on spray skirts, life jackets, and other accessories, see Chapter 14.

Manufacturer/model	Length (feet)	Width (inches)	Weight (pounds)	Material
Euro (1986)				
Breaker (wave ski)	8'	25½	26	polyethylene
Futura (1987)				
B-2 (surf ski)	19'	20	40	proprietary lay-up
Blade (surf ski)	19'6"	17½	40	proprietary lay-up
C-4 (surf ski)	20'	18	40	proprietary lay-up
Futura Series (surf ski)	15'-22'10"	20-24	35-65*	proprietary lay-up
Island (1987)				
Island Epoxy Double Wave Ski (tandem) (wave ski)	12'	32	32	fiberglass
Island Epoxy Fun Wave Ski (wave ski)	8'	27	28	fiberglass (chopper gun)
Island Epoxy Pro Wave Ski Series (wave ski)	7'8", 8'	22-27	12-18*	fiberglass
Karel's (1987)				
Cuda Ski (surf ski)	21'	18	30-35*	fiberglass (chopper gun) or Kevlar
Sea Horse (wave ski)	9'	30	32	fiberglass
Mega (1992)				
Jester Pro (surf ski)	11'6"	23	20	polyethylene
Jester Storm (surf ski)	11'6"	23	20	polyethylene
Jester Tico Series (surf ski)	11'6"	23	20	polyethylene
Jester Titan (surf ski)	11'6"	23	20	polyethylene
Ocean (1971)				
Sprinter (surf ski)	17'	21	50	polyethylene
Seda (1969)				
Surfer (wave ski)	8'	26	25	polyethylene
Twogood (1982)				
Chalup Ski (surf ski)	19'6"	17½	26-35*	fiberglass, Kevlar, or proprietary lay-up
Condore (tandem) (surf ski)	23'8"	20	43-55*	fiberglass, Kevlar, or proprietary lay-up
Mako (surf ski)	21'2"	15	27-35*	fiberglass, Kevlar, or proprietary lay-up
Offshore Series (surf ski)	18'4"	19	27-49*	fiberglass, Kevlar, or proprietary lay-up
Portlock (surf ski)	18'11"	18	25-33*	fiberglass, Kevlar, or proprietary lay-up
Predator II (surf ski)	19'4"	17	24-32*	fiberglass, Kevlar, or polyethylene
Valhalla (1983)				
Valhalla (surf ski)	19'	19¾	35	fiberglass
Victory Series (surf ski)	19'5"	18¼	30	fiberglass
Viking International (surf ski)	19'	19¼	32	fiberglass
Venturesport (1983)				
Crosstrainer (surf ski)	20'"	17½	35	fiberglass
Dolphin (surf ski)	19'	19	39	fiberglass or Kevlar
Needle (surf ski)	20'10"	15½	22-30*	fiberglass or Kevlar
Shearwater (surf ski)	20'6"	18	26-33*	fiberglass or Kevlar
Stinger LS (surf ski)	19'	19	35	fiberglass
West Side (1977)				
Wave Exceed (surf ski)	19'4"	18	28	Kevlar
Wave-Piercer (surf ski)	17'	20	27	Kevlar
Wave Ultra (surf ski)	19'	18	28	Kevlar
Wave XL (surf ski)	19'	18	28	Kevlar
X-Par Missile (surf ski)	23'	18	28	Kevlar

(Year in parentheses is year the company began making boats)
*Depending on model, material, or options

Keel	Bottom	Sides	Price (dollars)
straight with rise at ends	flat	straight	600
extreme rocker	deep V	flared	1200
moderate rocker	shallow V	straight	1600
extreme rocker	shallow arch	flared	1700
moderate rocker	shallow V	flared	1100-2250*
extreme rocker	shallow V	straight	1400
moderate rocker	shallow V	straight	600
moderate rocker	shallow V	straight	850
moderate rocker	round V or flat	straight	1700-2300*
straight with rise at ends	flat	straight	600
straight	shallow arch	tumblehome	900
straight	shallow arch	tumblehome	900
straight	shallow arch	tumblehome	900
straight	shallow arch	tumblehome	900
straight	shallow arch	tumblehome	900-1000*
extreme rocker	flat	straight	500
moderate rocker	shallow arch	straight	1050-1850*
moderate rocker	shallow arch	straight	1050-1850*
straight with rise at ends	flat	flared	1050-1850*
moderate rocker	shallow arch	straight	1050-1850*
moderate rocker	shallow arch	flared	1050-1850*
moderate rocker	shallow arch	straight	1050-1850*
moderate rocker	shallow arch	straight	1100
moderate rocker	shallow V	straight	1650-2000*
moderate rocker	rounded V	straight	2000
straight with rise at ends	shallow arch	straight	1500
moderate rocker	shallow arch	straight	1400
straight	shallow arch	straight	1650-2050*
straight with rise at ends	shallow arch	straight	1450-2050*
moderate rocker	shallow arch	straight	1450
moderate rocker	rounded V	flared	1800
moderate rocker	rounded V	flared	1800
moderate rocker	rounded V	flared	1800
moderate rocker	rounded V	flared	1800
moderate rocker	rounded V	flared	2000

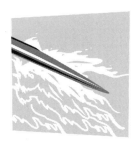

Chapter 10
Sit-on-top Kayaks

Not all kayaks have cockpits. A relatively new concept, the sit-on-top kayak, appeals to those who feel claustrophobic in an enclosed cockpit. If you miscalculate and dump over in a sit-on-top, so what? Just climb back aboard and continue paddling.

Most of the sit-on-tops have a shallow depression that you sit in and two small wells for your heels. A few even come with waterproof-fabric flaps that close around the paddler as a shelter from the weather.

The majority of sit-on-top designs are made for casual recreation, and are therefore quite stable. They're perfect for beginners, who find them less confining and intimidating than traditional decked models. Sit-on-tops are increasing in popularity, and even though the number of models is somewhat more limited than the conventional decked design, you shouldn't have any problem finding one that meets your needs.

The Builders

Among the manufacturers of sit-on-top kayaks are Hydra and Ocean, and some of their boats are discussed here. You'll find statistical details about sit-on-tops made by these and other manufacturers in the fact grids that follow this section.

Hydra

Hydra, of Knoxville, Tennessee, has been building boats since 1992. Its sit-on-tops are made of polyethylene.

The Adventurer, at 15 feet, 7 inches long, provides a removable, molded backrest for support. The self-bailing feature drains water at moderate cruising speeds through one-way valves on the bottom of the cockpit, saving the paddler from sitting in a puddle of water after the cockpit has emptied. The 50-pound Adventurer features a small, easy-to-reach port in the cockpit for storage of small items plus two optional larger hatches fore and aft. Price: $700.

The Aquanaut is the flagship of the Hydra line—a versatile 11-foot sit-on-top. It can be outfitted with 8-inch round hatches, full or half-back seats, and thigh straps. The keel is designed for good tracking, and its 30-inch width promotes stability. The seat is higher than the foot well for increased comfort, improved paddling position, and a drier ride. Price: $550.

The Aquanaut Twin, at a length of 13 feet, 9 inches, is the tandem version of the Aquanaut. Like the Aquanaut, the Twin has seats set higher than the foot well for comfort and a drier ride. Price: $600.

Ocean

Ocean Kayak, based in Ferndale, Washington, has been building boats since 1971. Its sit-on-tops are made of polyethylene.

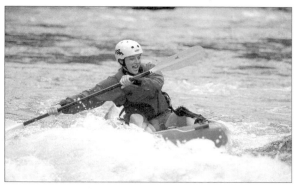

Riding the waves in a Torrent (courtesy Perception)

The Dawn Trakker (11 feet, 6 inches) is a blend of the sit-on-top and the traditional kayak, good for day cruising and light trips. Its size and flotation accommodate larger paddlers and payload. Molded-in tie-down and safety-line strap eyes add to the finishing details. Weight is 50 pounds. Price: $600–$700.

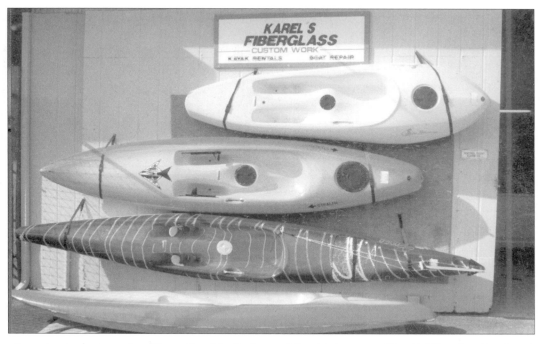

From top to bottom: Sea Horse, Stealth, Rodeo and Stealth (courtesy Karel's Fiberglass Products)

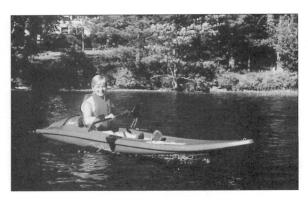

Typhoon (courtesy Old Town Canoe Co.)

The Pocket Trakker, at only 8 feet long, includes the design features of the longer Dawn Trakker in a compact boat. The short length makes it a good candidate for smaller people, including children. Price: $500–$550.

Compact and stable with a center keel

for tracking, the 9-foot-long Frenzy is recommended by Ocean Kayak for both beginners and experts. The short length makes for easy maneuvering on waves. The small size and good stability also provide a boat that can be used by children for flat-water lake cruising. Weight is 45 pounds. Price: about $400.

The 12-foot Malibu Two can be paddled as a one-person boat or as a tandem, with a center seat-well designed for a single paddler, pet, or small child. This 61-pound boat is a good day-tripping boat for families, fishing, or bird-watching. Price: $600–$700.

The Scrambler, at 11 feet, 2 inches, is used for surfing or cruising, and as a platform for diving or fishing. The Scrambler is available with stern storage space that can

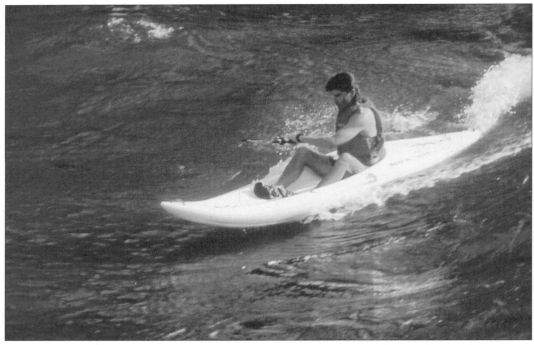

Spirit (courtesy Old Town Canoe Co.)

accommodate a small ice chest or a scuba unit. Weight is 45 pounds. Price: $500–$600.

The 12-foot Scrambler XT, at 56 pounds, is slightly wider and has a lower center of gravity than the Scrambler, making it an even better platform for diving. The enlarged back tank-well area handles a full scuba unit. The flatter bottom helps it perform as a surf boat, but it's also recommended for fishing and flatwater cruising. Price: $550–$600.

The 14-foot Scupper Classic is offered as a good choice for beginners who plan to paddle on calm to moderate water. The boat promises good tracking, but with enough rocker to permit easy turning without a rudder. Splash rails add lift and reduce spray. Price: $600.

The Scupper Pro, at 14 feet, 9 inches, can be outfitted with two large hatches that provide storage for tents, packs, extra paddles, dry bags, and scuba tanks. The boat is offered for long-distance paddling and exploration. Price: $750–$1000.

The 17-foot Sprinter was designed by

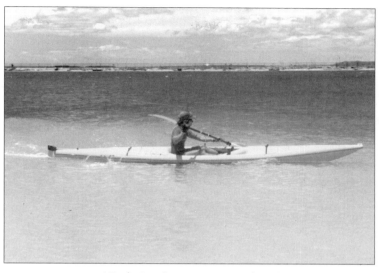

'Cuda Single (courtesy Karel's Fiberglass Products)

Tim Niemier and two-time Olympic gold medalist Greg Barton with speed and acceleration in mind. The goal was maximum length and minimum width for high performance. Price: $900–$1000.

Tim Niemier designed the 10-foot, 5-inch Yahoo!, a sit-on-top river kayak. A low center of gravity and good stability help movement through the waves, while its rocker promotes maneuverability. Not limited to rivers, it can also be used for surfing. Price: $450–$500.

Sit-on-top Kayaks

The following grids present details on the lineup of sit-on-top kayaks offered by selected manufacturers. See the end of this chapter for the addresses and phone numbers of these and other manufacturers. For information on paddles, see Chapter 3. For information on spray skirts, life jackets, and other accessories, see Chapter 14.

Manufacturer/model	Length (feet)	Width (inches)	Weight (pounds)	Material
Competition (1996)				
CK 3.4	13'5"	25	40	polyethylene
CK 4.2	13'5"	24	43	polyethylene
CK 4.4	17'4"	26	50	polyethylene
Dagger (1988)				
Cayman (casual recreation)	12'4"	29	55	polyethylene
Frolic	10'	30	48	polyethylene
Pegasus	10'6"	31	48	polyethylene
Tiki (tandem)	13'	32	66	polyethylene
Easy Rider (1970)				
Cub Scout Multi-Use	12'6"	35	45-55*	fiberglass or Kevlar
Englehart (1988)				
Epibrat (designed for children)	9'8"	23	35	polyethylene
Epitot (designed for children)	5'9"	21	24	polyethylene
Futura (1987)				
Futura (surf ski)	15'	24	35	proprietary lay-up
Futura II (surf ski)	19'	20	35	proprietary lay-up
Futura TS (surf ski)	20'	23	60	proprietary lay-up
Spear (casual recreation)	16'	19	35	proprietary lay-up
Glenwa (1992)				
Cobra Explorer	13'5"	31	43	polyethylene
Cobra Play	12'1"	27	38	polyethylene
Cobra Tandem	15'	36	57	polyethylene
Cobra XL	13'9"	28½	43	polyethylene
Hobie Cat (1968)				
Odyssey (tandem) (casual recreation)	14'	33	80	polyethylene
Pursuit (casual recreation)	12'	28	47	polyethylene
Hop on Top (1995)				
12' HopOnTop (casual recreation)	12'	27	32	fiberglass
16' HopOnTop (sea touring)	16'	27	39-45*	fiberglass or Kevlar
18' HopOnTop (sea touring)	18'3"	24	40-48*	fiberglass or Kevlar
Hydra (1992)				
Adventurer (casual recreation)	15'7"	24	50	polyethylene
Aquanaut (casual recreation)	11'	30	42	polyethylene
AquanautTwin (tandem) (casual recreation)	13'9"	30	60	polyethylene
Janautica/Splashdance (1983)				
Simon-PO (casual recreation)	13'9"	25	50	polyethylene
Karel's (1987)				
Cuda Double	18'	28	65	fiberglass
Cuda Single	16'	24	38	fiberglass
Dolphin	14'	30	51	proprietary lay-up
Rodeo	14'	28	36	fiberglass
Spike	12'	30	48	proprietary lay-up
Stealth	12'	30	38	fiberglass
Kiwi (1988)				
Sea Vu (casual recreation)	8'11"	25	38	polyethylene
Tad Kat (casual recreation)	8'11"	25	79	polyethylene
Tadpole II (casual recreation)	8'11"	25	37	polyethylene

Keel	Bottom	Sides	Price (dollars)
straight with rise at ends	shallow arch	flared	715
straight with rise at ends	shallow arch	flared	525
straight with rise at ends	shallow arch	flared	729
moderate rocker	shallow arch	flared	600
straight with rise at ends	shallow arch	straight	500
moderate rocker	shallow arch	tumblehome	600
straight with rise at ends	shallow arch	straight	700
moderate rocker	shallow V	flared	1700-2400*
straight with rise at ends	deep V	straight	250
straight with rise at ends	deep arch	straight	200
moderate rocker	shallow V	flared	1100
straight with rise at ends	rounded V	flared	1350
moderate rocker	rounded V	flared	1950
extreme rocker	shallow arch	flared	1150
straight with rise at ends	shallow arch	straight	455
moderate rocker	shallow V	straight	400
straight with rise at ends	deep V	straight	700
straight with rise at ends	shallow arch	straight	510
moderate rocker	rounded V	straight	750
moderate rocker	rounded V	straight	600
moderate rocker	shallow arch	straight	1000
moderate rocker	shallow arch	straight	1700-2100*
straight with rise at ends	rounded V	straight	1900-2300*
straight with rise at ends	rounded V	straight	700
straight with rise at ends	deep V	flared	550
straight with rise at ends	shallow V	flared	600
straight with rise at ends	shallow arch V	tumblehome	500
moderate rocker	shallow arch	flared	1500
moderate rocker	shallow arch	flared	1200
moderate rocker	rounded V	straight	900
moderate rocker	rounded V	flared	1100
moderate rocker	rounded V	straight	800
moderate rocker	rounded V	straight	950
straight with rise at ends	flat	tumblehome	500
straight with rise at ends	flat	tumblehome	1000
straight with rise at ends	flat	tumblehome	450

Manufacturer/model	Length (feet)	Width (inches)	Weight (pounds)	Material
Mainstream (1996)				
Jazz (casual recreation)	9'	30	35	polyethylene
Tango (casual recreation)	12'	34	52	polyethylene
Necky (1983)				
Dorado	11'	29	45	polyethylene
Santa Cruze (tandem)	13'	31	60	polyethylene
Ocean (1971)				
Dawn Trakker	11'6"	28	50	polyethylene
Malibu Two (tandem)	12'	34	61	polyethylene
Pocket Trakker	8'	32	40	polyethylene
Scrambler Series	11'2', 12'	28, 29	45-56*	polyethylene
Scupper Classic	14'	26	48	polyethylene
Scupper Pro Series	14'9"	26	55	polyethylene
Sprinter	17'	21	48	polyethylene
Super Frenzy	9'3"	30	45	polyethylene
Yahoo!	10'5"	30	53	polyethylene
Yak Board	8'	29	40	polyethylene
Zest Two (tandem)	16'	32	68	polyethylene
Old Town (1898)				
Dimension Solo (casual recreation)	13'2"	30½	44	polyethylene
Dimension Spirit (casual recreation)	11'	28	35	polyethylene
Sandpiper (casual recreation)	9'6"	28½	35	polyethylene
Spirit Duo (tandem)				
(casual recreation)	15'2"	34½	75	polyethylene
Typhoon (casual recreation)	11'2"	29½	39	polyethylene
Perception (1975)				
Aquaterra Prism (sea touring)	14'2"	27	58	polyethylene
Aquaterra Swing (sea touring)	13'3"	31	58	polyethylene
Aquaterra Synchro (tandem)				
(sea touring)	15'7"	34	84	polyethylene
Torrent Series (whitewater)	8'2", 8'11"	24½	36-40*	polyethylene
Prijon (1985)				
Twister Premier (whitewater)	10'2"	25	35	polyethylene
Pyranha (1974)				
Surf Jet 305	10'1"	24	45	polyethylene
Seda (1969)				
Revenge (sea touring)	16'6"	25	39-54	fiberglass or Kevlar
Tsunami (1986)				
X-O Crossover	12'6"	24	40	Kevlar
X-1 Rocket	16'	20½	50	Kevlar
X-2 Starship	19'10"	29	90	Kevlar
X-7 Mojo	10'7"	23	35	Kevlar
X-15 Scramjet	14'	23	40	Kevlar
Venturesport (1983)				
Freedom	17'2"	25	53	fiberglass
Wilderness Systems (1986)				
Riot (casual touring)	9'8"	30	38	polyethylene
Two-Can (tandem)				
(casual recreation)	15'6"	27	57	polyethylene

(Year in parentheses is year the company began making boats)
*Depending on model, material, or options

Keel	Bottom	Sides	Price (dollars)
moderate rocker	shallow arch	straight	350
moderate rocker	shallow arch	straight	500
moderate rocker	shallow V	straight	500
moderate rocker	shallow V	straight	700
moderate rocker	deep V	flared	600-700*
moderate rocker	deep V	straight	600-700*
moderate rocker	deep V	flared	500-550*
moderate rocker	deep V	straight	500-600*
moderate rocker	deep V	straight	600
moderate rocker	deep V	straight	750-1000*
straight ends	shallow arch	tumblehome	900-1000*
moderate rocker	deep V	straight	400-450
extreme rocker	shallow arch	tumblehome	450-500*
straight with rise at ends	shallow V	flared	300-350
moderate rocker	deep V	straight	650-800*
straight with rise at ends	shallow arch	tumblehome	450
straight with rise at ends	flat	tumblehome	400
straight with rise at ends	shallow V	tumblehome	300
straight with rise at ends	flat	tumblehome	600
straight with rise at ends	flat	tumblehome	450
straight with rise at ends	flat	straight	600
straight with rise at ends	shallow arch	flared	650
straight with rise at ends	shallow arch	flared	750
extreme rocker	flat	straight	450-550
extreme rocker	flat	flared	600
moderate rocker	shallow arch	flared	650
straight with rise at ends	shallow V	flared	900-1300*
extreme rocker	shallow arch	tumblehome	1500
extreme rocker	shallow V	flared	2500
moderate rocker	shallow V	flared	3500
extreme rocker	shallow arch	flared	1500
extreme rocker	shallow arch	tumblehome	2500
straight with rise at ends	shallow arch	flared	1350
moderate rocker	shallow arch	tumblehome	450
straight with rise at ends	shallow arch	tumblehome	650

Sit-on-top Kayak Manufacturers

Competition Kayak
    P.O. Box 31064
    Albuquerque, NM 87190
    (505) 888–5800
    Fax (505) 888–7912

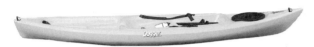

Dagger Canoe Co.'s Cayman

Dagger Canoe Company
P.O. Box 1500
Harriman, TN 37748
(423) 882–0404
Fax (423) 882–8153

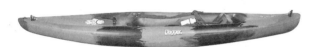

Dagger Canoe Co.'s Pegasus

Easy Rider Canoe & Kayak Company
    P.O. Box 88108
    Seattle, WA 98138
    (425) 228–3633
    Fax (425) 277–8778

Englehart Products Inc. (EPI)
    P.O. Box 377
    Newbury, OH 44065
    (216) 564–5565
    Fax (216) 564–5515

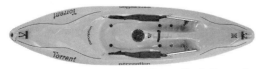

Perception's Torrent

Futura Surf Skis
    730 West 19th Street
    National City, CA 91950
    (619) 474–8382
    Fax (619) 474–5167

Glenwa
    P.O. Box 3134
    Gardena, CA 90247
    (310) 327–9216
    Fax (310) 327–8952
    E-mail: cobrakayaks@worldnet.att.net
    Web: http://www.cobrakayaks.com

Hobie Cat Company
    4925 Oceanside Boulevard
    Oceanside, CA 92056
    (760) 758–9100 ext. 400
    Fax (760) 758–1841

Hop On Top Kayaks
    P.O. Box 139
    Jamestown, RI 02835
    (401) 423–1815
    Fax (401) 423–1815

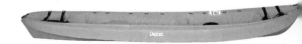

Wilderness System's Two-can

Hydra Kayaks
    5061 South National Drive
    Knoxville, TN 37914
    (800) 537–8888
    Fax (305) 836–1296

Janautica/Splashdance
    Highway 85 South
    Niceville, FL 32578

(850) 678–1637
Fax (850) 678–1637

Karel's Fiberglass Products
789 Kailua Road
Kailua HI 96734
(808) 261–8424
Fax (808) 261–8424

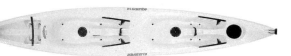

Perception's Synchro

Kiwi Kayak Company
2454 Vista Del Monte
Concord, CA 94520
(510) 692–2041
Fax (510) 692–2042

Mainstream Products
182 Kayaker Way
Easley, SC 29642
(864) 859–9933
Fax (864) 859–9977

Necky Kayaks
1100 Riverside Road
Abbotsford, British Columbia V2S
7P1
(604) 850–1206
Fax (604) 850–3197

Ocean Kayak
P.O. Box 5003
Ferndale, WA 98248
(800) 852–9257
Fax (360) 366–2628

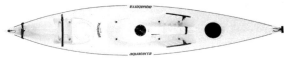

Perception's Swing

Old Town Canoe Company
58 Middle Street
Old Town, ME 04468
(207) 827–5513
Fax (207) 827–2779

Perception, Inc.
P.O. Box 8002
Easley, SC 29641
(803) 859–7518
Fax (803) 855–5995

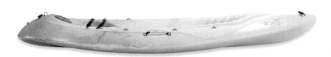

Wilderness Systems' Riot

Prijon/Wildwasser Sport USA
P.O. Box 4617
Boulder, CO 80306
(303) 444–2336
Fax (303) 444–2375

Pyranha/Impex International
1107 Station Road
Bellport, NY 11713
(513) 286–1988

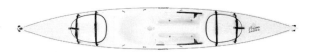

Perception's Prism

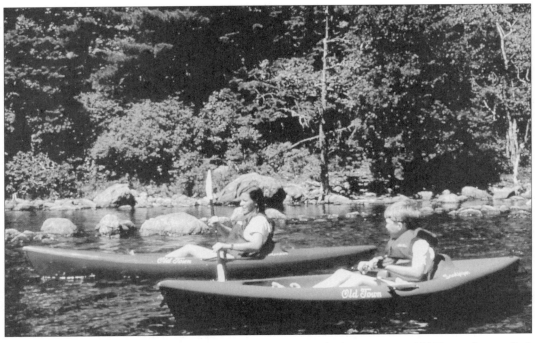

Sandpiper (courtesy Old Town Canoe Co.)

Seda Products
    926 Coolidge Avenue
    National City, CA 91950
    (619) 336–2444
    Fax (619) 336–2405

Tsunami
    13732 Bear Mountain Road
    Redding, CA 96003
    (916) 275–4313
    Fax (916) 275–3090

Venturesport Kayaks & Surf Skis
    P.O. Box 610145
    Miami, FL 33261
    (561) 395–1376

Wilderness Systems
    P.O. Box 4339
    Archdale, NC 27263
    (910) 434–7470
    Fax (910) 434–6912

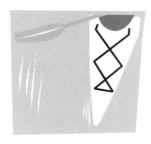

Chapter 11
Folding Kayaks

Folding kayaks were first developed at the turn of the twentieth century by a German tailor named Hans Klepper, who wanted to take a boat on crowded trains to reach the lakes and rivers of Europe. The folding kayak—consisting of a collapsible frame covered by fabric—was born, and the idea now appeals to the modern air traveler and apartment dweller.

Disassembled, a folding boat fits into two or three duffels that can be checked as luggage or stored in a closet. These boats are slightly less responsive than hard-shell kayaks, and they can be very expensive, but for portability, nothing can beat them. (See the end of this chapter for information on another type of portable boat, the take-apart kayak.)

The Klepper Resume

The following expeditions have used Klepper folding kayaks, an impressive list indeed:

1909 C. E. Layton: paddled across the English Channel
1923 Karl Schott: kayaked by sea from Germany to India
1926 Roald Amundsen: North Pole expedition
1928 Admiral Byrd: South Pole expedition
1928 Capt. Romer: crossed the Atlantic Ocean
1928 Sven Hedin: Asian explorations
1935 Dr. Sorge: Spitzbergen expedition
1954 H. Rittlinger: Upper Nile and Sudan
1955 Hans Ertl: Andes-Amazon expedition
1956 Dr. Hannes Lindemann: sailed across the Atlantic
1970 John Dowd: kayaked from Singapore to Australia
1978 K. Gallei: east coast of Greenland
1979 Charles Porter: sculled around Cape Horn
1983 Kimmich and Eckstein: Marañón expedition
1984 Fuchs and Neuber: winter trip to Cape Horn

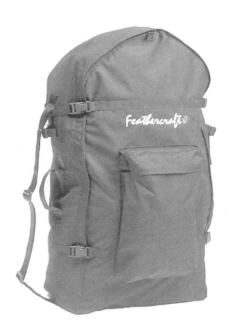

Feathercrafts's pack-bag for a single kayak

1985 Fuchs and Porter: magnetic North
   Pole
1987 Lindenkamp and Meyer: Tibet expedition
1989 Howard Rice: sailed solo around
   Cape Horn
1991 Gail Ferris: Point Barrow, Alaska;
   Arctic Ocean
1992 Stiller and Brown: semi-circumnaviga-
   tion of Australia

Proud Klepper owners have their own club: International Klepper Society, P.O. Box 973, Good Hart, MI 49737.

Good Read: Folding Kayaks

The Complete Folding Kayaker, by Ralph Diaz (Camden, Maine: Ragged Mountain Press, 1994), is the only book devoted solely to folding kayaks. Diaz is a very experienced proponent of the craft.

The Builders

Among the manufacturers of folding kayaks are Feathercraft and Klepper, and some of their boats are discussed here. You'll find statistical details on folding kayaks made by these and other manufacturers in the fact grids that follow this section.

Feathercraft

Feathercraft Products, of Vancouver, British Columbia, has been building folding kayaks since 1977. The kayaks' framework is made of aircraft-quality anodized aluminum tubing, shock-corded for ease of assembly. The cross-frames are injection-molded polycarbonate. The deck is made of heavy nylon fabric coated with urethane, and the hull is Hypalon-coated nylon.

The Klondike is the newest addition to the Feathercraft line. Its open-cockpit design can be configured as a single, a double, or even a triple, simply by moving deck bars and seating placement. The 17-foot, 10-inch boat accommodates gear storage for two weeks or more. The Klondike is shorter, lighter, and slightly easier to assemble than Feathercraft's K2 Expedition Double, and also carries less. Designed for the family, the Klondike is very stable. Price: $3900.

The updated KI Single Expedition now sports a graceful upswept bow for smoother water entry. There is an increased waterline and less bow wake, contributing to improved speed and surfing ability. The pro-

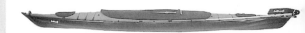

Feathercraft's Klondike

118

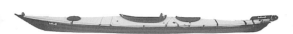

Feathercraft's K1 Expedition Single

nounced V-shaped hull of this large-volume single makes for good tracking. Hatches are located in the bow and stern, and internal air sponsons tension the skin to help ensure stability. Standard accessories include adjustable padded seat, flip-up surf rudder, perimeter deck-lines, and cross-deck tie-downs, travel-style pack-bag, nylon spray skirt, sea sock, and repair kit. Price: $3800.

The K2 Expedition Double, at 19 feet, 3 inches long, is a high-volume double kayak designed for maximum storage capacity. Bow and stern hatches make for easy access to storage space that can handle the gear and supplies for a multi-week camping trip. An upswept bow allows for a drier ride, and the wide beam and internal air sponsons provide stability. Padded sling-style seats are adjustable, and the low-profile cockpit coaming allows use of individual sea socks without inhibiting paddling. The K2 packs into either one bag or two. The Double comes with a long list of standard accessories. Price: $4600.

The K Light Plus, at 12 feet, 10 inches, is a low-maintenance kayak good for day trips or long weekends. The design incorporates good rocker with a defined keel, so it tracks well. A rudder is available as an option. Price: $1800.

The design of the Khatsalano (17 feet, 9 inches) is derived from the traditional Greenland kayaks of the Inuit people and is known for speed, performance, and maneuverability. Small-diameter sponsons

have been added to the Khatsalano, rounding out the chines and adding stability. This design allows you to choose whether to inflate the sponsons or not, depending on the water you're paddling that day. As with all Feathercraft models, the Khatsalano comes with an array of standard accessories. Price: $3800–$3950.

Klepper

Klepper Folding Kayaks is the German company that, in 1907, invented the folding kayak. Its office in the United States is located in Sacramento, California. Klep-

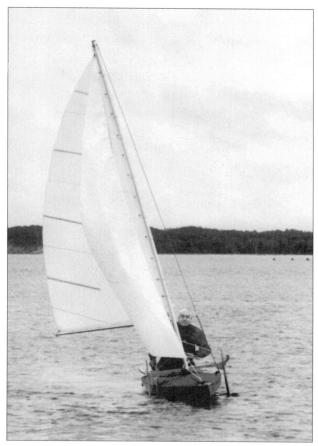

Seavivor folding kayak with a Marconi sailing rig (courtesy Seavivor)

Journeys in Folding Kayaks

The ambitious journeys taken in folding kayaks have resulted in some excellent books.

Happy Isles of Oceania, by Paul Theroux (New York: Ballentine Books, 1993): a highly literate and personal account of an ambitious paddling tour of the South Pacific islands.

A Boat in Our Baggage: Around the World with a Kayak, by Maria Coffey (Camden, Maine: Ragged Mountain Press, 1995): an around-the-world romp by a husband-and-wife team on a budget vacation filled with close encounters with the locals they meet along the way.

Alone at Sea, by Hannes Lindemann (Somerset, California: Western Folding Kayak Center): the classic, and very understated, account of a 72-day solo crossing of the Atlantic in 1956.

Yukon Summer, by Eugene Cantin (Chronicle Books, 1973): long out-of-print but a fine read; the story of a young man's solo cruise through the Canada-Alaska wilderness in a Klepper kayak. Cantin had very little experience before setting off, making his story even more compelling.

pers, while expensive, are known for high quality. The framework is made of solid mountain ash, with birch plywood ribs and floorboards, and the parts are color- and number-coded for assembly. The decks are made of canvas and the hulls are Hypalon-coated canvas.

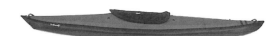

Feathercraft's KLight Kayak

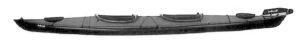

Feathercraft's K2 Expedition Double

The Aerius 2000, 12½ feet long, is a versatile boat with sufficient space to handle luggage for longer weekends and for trips on rivers or lakes. The 2000 comes with deck load tie-downs, paddle holder, bow and stern fittings, contoured cushioned seat, and a swivel backrest. It also includes a mast step, mast support bracket, and rudder bracket to accommodate three different sails. Price: $2350.

The Aerius Classic Single provides storage capacity for extended trips on lakes, open rivers, and the ocean. The boat is cred-

ited with speed, good tracking, and stability. A specially designed rudder helps turn the kayak into a smooth-performing sailboat. The 15-foot Classic comes with bow and stern fittings, contoured cushioned seat with swivel backrest, plus the mast step, mast support bracket, and rudder bracket to accommodate any of the four Klepper sails. Price: $2800. Klepper offers its Aerius Classic Double (tandem) at $3200.

The Aerius Expedition Single, at a length of 15 feet, builds upon the proven Aerius Classic design. The Expedition Single offers a strong hull and keel-strip reinforcement for protection against rock, ice, or coral. Available in four colors, from signal red to camouflage olive. Price: $3400. Klepper offers its Aerius Expedition Double (tandem) at $4000.

The Aerius Quattro XT, a tandem

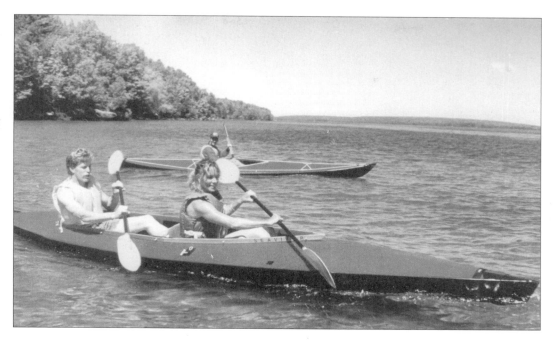

Seavivor's Classic Double (front) and Greenland Solo (courtesy Seavivor)

model, is the only kayak in the world with an adjustable hull. The Quattro XT has four fully integrated air sponsons for increased loading capacity and buoyancy. Through variable inflation of the upper and lower sponsons, the hull shape can be changed from V to U, enabling heavy loads to be carried through shallow water. The hardwood frame is available in black or natural color. The length is 17 feet, and weight is 82 pounds. Price: $4900.

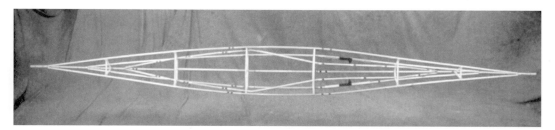

Feathercraft's Khatsalano framework

Folding Kayaks

The following grids present details on the lineup of folding kayaks offered by selected manufacturers. At the end of the grids are the addresses and phone numbers of these and other manufacturers. For information on paddles, see Chapter 3. For information on spray skirts, life jackets, and other accessories, see Chapter 14.

Manufacturer/model	Length (feet)	Width (inches)	Weight (pounds)	Material
Feathercraft (1977)				
Khatsalano Series	17'9"	22-23½	43-45*	anodized aluminum tubing injection-molded polycarbonate urethane-coated nylon Hypalon-coated nylon
K1 Expedition Single	15'11"	25	55	anodized aluminum tubing injection-molded polycarbonate urethane-coated nylon Hypalon-coated nylon
K2 Expedition Double	19'3"	33	87	anodized aluminum tubing injection-molded polycarbonate urethane-coated nylon Hypalon-coated nylon
K Light Plus	12'10"	25	33	anodized aluminum tubing injection-molded polycarbonate urethane-coated nylon Hypalon-coated nylon
Koho Expedition Single	11'6"	22	28	anodized aluminum tubing injection-molded polycarbonate urethane-coated nylon Hypalon-coated nylon
Klondike	17'10"	25	63	anodized aluminum tubing injection-molded polycarbonate urethane-coated nylon Hypalon-coated nylon
S.T. Expedition	13'6"	27	48	anodized aluminum tubing injection-molded polycarbonate urethane-coated nylon Hypalon-coated nylon
Folbot (1933)				
Aleut	12'	29	38	anodized aluminum tubing acrylic-coated poly/cotton Hypalon-coated nylon
Greenland II	17'	34	64	anodized aluminum tubing glass-filled polycarbonate acrylic-coated poly/cotton Hypalon-coated nylon
Jumbo/Pouch (1950)				
Pouch Fold-Boat FK-450	15'	26	46	solid mountain ash birch plywood canvas Hypalon-coated canvas
Pouch Fold-Boat FK-550	18'2"	34	66	solid mountain ash birch plywood Hypalon-coated canvas
Kayak Lab (1992)				
Sigma-1	14'7"	32	39	anodized aluminum tubing polyurethane-coated nylon
Sigma-2	17'4"	33	49	anodized aluminum tubing anodized aluminum tubing
Sigma-1-A	14'7"	26	39	polyurethane-coated nylon anodized aluminum tubing anodized aluminum tubing
Sigma-2-Z	17'4"	33	49	polyurethane-coated nylon anodized aluminum tubing anodized aluminum tubing polyurethane-coated nylon
Klepper (1907)				
Aerius Classic Single	15'	28	55	solid mountain ash birch plywood canvas Hypalon-coated canvas
Aerius Classic Double (tandem)	17'	34	71	solid mountain ash birch plywood canvas Hypalon-coated canvas
Aerius Expedition Single	15'	28	60	solid mountain ash birch plywood canvas Hypalon-coated canvas

Keel	Bottom	Sides	Price (dollars)
straight with rise at ends	shallow V	flared	3800-3950*
straight with rise at ends	shallow V	flared	3800
moderate rocker	shallow V	flared	4600
moderate rocker	shallow V	flared	1800
moderate rocker	shallow V	flared	1500
straight with rise at ends	shallow V	flared	3900
extreme rocker	shallow arch	tumblehome	3250
glass-filled polycarbonate			
straight	rounded V	flared	1200
straight	rounded V	flared	1800
straight	shallow V	flared	1500
canvas			
straight	shallow V	flared	1300
straight	shallow V	tumblehome	2200
straight	shallow V	tumblehome	3000
straight	shallow V	tumblehome	2200
straight	shallow V	tumblehome	3000
straight with rise at ends	shallow V	flared	2800
straight	rounded V	flared	3200
straight with rise at ends	shallow V	flared	3400

Manufacturer/model	Length (feet)	Width (inches)	Weight (pounds)	Material
Aerius Expedition Double (tandem)	17'	34	77	solid mountain ash birch plywood canvas Hypalon-coated canvas
Aerius Quattro XT (tandem)	17'	34	82	solid mountain ash birch plywood canvas Hypalon-coated canvas
Aerius 2000	12'6"	26	42	solid mountain ash birch plywood canvas Hypalon-coated canvas
Nautiraid (About 1956) Double Raid	16'6"	34	69	solid mountain ash birch plywood urethane-coated polyester Hypalon-coated nylon
Grand Raid	17'	36	77	solid mountain ash birch plywood urethane-coated polyester Hypalon-coated nylon
Miniraid	12'	26	37	solid mountain ash birch plywood urethane-coated polyester Hypalon-coated nylon
Raid 14	14'	25	45	solid mountain ash birch plywood urethane-coated polyester Hypalon-coated nylon
Single Raid	15'2"	26	48	solid mountain ash birch plywood urethane-coated polyester Hypalon-coated nylon
Touring Raid	15'	32	53	solid mountain ash birch plywood urethane-coated polyester Hypalon-coated nylon
Pouch Faltboote (1953) Eureka I	15'	26	48	solid ash birch plywood canvas urethane-coated poly/cotton
Eureka II	18'	34	72	solid ash birch plywood canvas urethane-coated poly/cotton
Seavivor (1977) Classic Double Series	17'	36	67-70*	solid ash birch plywood urethane-coated nylon
Greenland Solo	17'10"	24	52	solid ash birch plywood urethane-coated nylon
Tramper	13'6"	27	31	solid ash birch plywood urethane-coated nylon
Whale Craft (1949) Whalecraft Double (tandem)	17'	34	65	solid ash birch plywood urethane-coated nylon
Whalecraft Single	14'	30	55	solid ash birch plywood urethane-coated nylon

(Year in parentheses is year the company began making folding kayaks or other boats)
* Depending on model

Keel	Bottom	Sides	Price (dollars)
straight	rounded V	flared	4000
straight	rounded V	flared	4900
straight with rise at ends	shallow V	flared	2350
straight with rise at ends	shallow V	flared	2750
straight with rise at ends	shallow arch	flared	3000
moderate rocker	shallow arch	flared	1250
straight with rise at ends	shallow arch	flared	1850
straight with rise at ends	shallow V	flared	2150
straight with rise at ends	shallow arch	flared	1850
straight	shallow V	flared	1850
straight	shallow V	flared	2000
straight	shallow arch	flared	3850-4200*
straight with rise at ends	rounded V	flared	3400
extreme rocker	shallow V	flared	2900
moderate rocker	shallow arch	flared	2300
extreme rocker	rounded V	flared	1900

Manufacturers of Folding Kayaks

Feathercraft Products
#4-1244 Cartwright Street
Vancouver, British Columbia V6H 3R8
(604) 681–8437

Folbot
P.O. Box 70877
Charleston, SC 29415
(800) 533–5099

Kayak Lab
18 Regina Drive
Chelmsford, MA 01824
(978) 256–5515
Fax (978) 256–5515

Klepper Folding Kayaks
100 Cadillac Drive, Suite 117
Sacramento, CA 95825
(800) 323–3525
Web: http://www.klepper.com

Nautiraid Folding Kayaks
Seda Products
926 Coolidge Avenue
National City, CA 91950
(619) 336–2444

Commando Kayaks

The incredible—and true—story of Australian commandos in kayaks blowing up ships in Singapore during World War II can be found in *The Heroes,* by Ronald McKee (New York: Harcourt Brace, 1960).

If this story appeals, you should also try *Cockleshell Heroes,* by Cecil Phillips (London: Hinneman, 1957), about a group of iron-nerved kayakers doing the same thing in occupied France. Long out-of-print, these books can still be found in libraries or through interlibrary loan.

Pouch Faltboote
6155 Mt. Auburn Road
Somerset, CA 95684-0130
(916) 626–8647
Fax (916) 626–6893

Seavivor Folding Boats
576 Arlington Avenue
Des Plaines, IL 60016
(847) 297–5953
Web: http://www.seavivor.com

Whale Craft Folding Kayaks
4011 Fremont
Seattle, WA 98103
(206) 634–0628
Fax (206) 223–0399

Special Resources

The Western Folding Kayak Center makes side-by-side comparison of various models easier by displaying the wares of five manufacturers in one location: Feathercraft, Folbot, Klepper, Nautiraid, and Pouch. The center is at 6155 Mt. Aukum Road, Somerset, CA 95684 (530–626–8647).

Two companies that rent folding kayaks to people setting out for far-flung destinations are Folding Kayak Adventures, P.O. Box 51008, Seattle, WA 98115 (800-586-9318) and Baidarka Boats, Box 6001, Sitka, AK (907–747–8996).

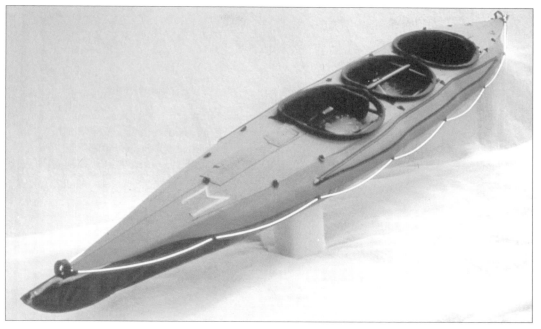

Sigma 2-Z (courtesy Kayak Lab)

Take-Apart Kayaks

To deal with the problems of portability of
rigid boats, kayak designers have come up
with an ingenious idea: a kayak that breaks
down into either two, three, or four parts
and is then reassembled at the put-in. If you
need portability in a touring kayak but
prefer a rigid boat over a folding model,
these are the boats for you.

Manufacturers of Take-Apart Kayaks

Ainsworth
  P.O. Box 207
  Norwich, VT 05055
  (802) 649–2952
  Fax (802) 649–2254

Easy Rider Canoe & Kayak Company
  P.O. Box 88108
  Seattle, WA 98138
  (425) 228–3633
  Fax (425) 277–8778

Take-Apart Kayaks

The following grids present details on the lineup of take-apart kayaks offered by Ainsworth
and Easy Rider.

Manufacturer/model	Length (feet)	Width (inches)	Weight (pounds)	Material
Ainsworth (1970)				
Horizon 3	16'	24	55	proprietary lay-up
Easy Rider (1970)				
Beluga 2-Piece Take-A-Part	16'8"	32	58-65*	fiberglass or Kevlar
Eskimo 15 CRX 2-Piece Take-A-Part	15'	24½	46-51*	fiberglass or Kevlar
Eskimo 17 CRX 3-Piece Take-A-Part	17'	24½	55	Kevlar
Eskimo 22-6 CRX 2-Piece Take-A-Part	22'6"	29	88-98*	fiberglass or Kevlar
Eskimo 22-6 CRX 4-Piece Take-A-Part	22'6"	29	98	Kevlar

(Year in parentheses is year the company began making boats)
* Depending on model, material, or options

Keel	Bottom	Sides	Price (dollars)
straight with rise at ends	shallow V	tumblehome	1500
straight with rise at ends	shallow arch	flared	2400-3200*
straight with rise at ends	shallow V	flared	2700-3200*
straight with rise at ends	shallow V	flared	3900
straight with rise at ends	shallow V	flared	4600-5500*
straight with rise at ends	shallow V	flared	6500

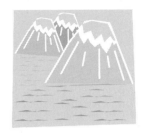

Chapter 12
Inflatable Kayaks

The modern inflatable kayaks, with their new and improved materials and designs, offer advantages over more traditional hardshell boats. For one thing, they are considerably easier for beginners because they're much more stable, and it isn't necessary to learn the Eskimo roll. They are more forgiving when they hit a rock because they tend to bounce off it. They are a little sluggish in flat stretches of a river, but the more expensive models are rigid and solve much of that problem. The greatest advantage of an inflatable kayak is its compactness when deflated. They are easy to transport in the trunk of your car, and they can be checked as regular luggage on an airline flight.

The most recent versions of inflatable kayaks include not only those made for whitewater but those made for sea kayaking and playboating. With self-bailing bottoms and intricate curves, today's inflatable kayaks have very few drawbacks for a boat that was once routinely ridiculed.

Design

The designs of inflatable boats are more limited than those of hardshell boats made of plastic or fiberglass; there are nonetheless a surprising number of differences between models. Besides the obvious differences in length and width, inflatable kayaks can vary in the amount of bow and stern lift and the shape of the tubes themselves. The placement of seats and air valves are variables, too.

Design is important because it determines how the boat will handle. Other features, such as the number of air chambers, affect safety as well.

Size

A one-person inflatable kayak typically ranges in size from 9 to 10½ feet, and a two-person model, from 11 to 12½ feet. Kayaks designed for sea touring are much longer.

The larger models can carry more gear,

but they're harder to maneuver because they respond more slowly. A larger boat is more stable in ocean waves or whitewater—but if you're looking for more excitement, you might want a smaller boat. Smaller boats displace less water, so they're more suitable for shallow streams.

Bow and Stern Lift

An upturned bow and stern provide easier turning and are useful in keeping water out of the boat. But too much upturn can create problems: The amount of gear you can store on boat is reduced; large waves have a greater ability to stop the boat; and a wind blowing upstream can bring your forward progress to a standstill.

Tube Size

The size of the boat's tubes influences the boat's handling and the amount of water that gets into the boat. On boats that aren't self-bailing (see the discussion of self-bailing below), a larger tube reduces the amount of water entering the boat. Since the added weight of water makes a boat difficult to handle, the greater flotation afforded by the larger tubes can be an important safety factor. The added flotation also allows more gear to be taken. Tube size influences maneuverability, however, since a larger tube is more sluggish and requires more effort to move.

Rigidity

A boat's rigidity is an important aspect of its design. Generally, a rigid boat is more maneuverable because it skims across the top of the water more easily. The self-bailing floors now used in inflatable kayaks, especially the closed-cell foam floors, offer a more rigid boat. A few kayakers, though, prefer a more flexible boat in whitewater because its loose design conforms to the water as it moves through the waves, providing more stability.

Materials

Most high-quality inflatables have either a nylon or polyester fabric base with a protective coating that makes the fabric airtight and resists abrasion. The more durable coatings include neoprene, Hypalon, PVC (polyvinyl chloride), and polyurethane. Technical terms such as "tensile strength" and "tear strength" are used to describe these materials, but ultimately the safest bet to find a good quality boat is to buy from a top-quality manufacturer.

Self Bailers

One of the greatest improvements in inflatable kayaks has been the self-bailing floor. As its name implies, it allows water to escape through the bottom of the boat and into the river, lake, or ocean, usually through holes in the floor near the tubes. Most of the floors are either inflatable or made of closed-cell foam.

A self-bailing boat not only eliminates the tedium of bailing but also improves safety, because a water-laden boat is heavy

Good Reads: Inflatable Kayaks

The Complete Inflatable Kayaker, by Jeff Bennett (Camden, Maine: Ragged Mountain Press, 1996)

Inflatable Kayaking: The Complete Guide, by Cecil Kuhne (Mechanicsburg, Pennsylvania: Stackpole Books, 1997)

and difficult to maneuver, increasing the possibility of colliding sideways on a boulder in whitewater. The self-bailing option, however, is an expensive one, and the additional material can add weight and bulk to a kayak. Some kayakers believe that self-bailing boats are more prone to flipping in whitewater because the added flotation causes the boat to ride higher on the water.

The Builders

Among the manufacturers of inflatable kayaks are AIRE and Jumbo, and some of their boats are discussed here. You'll find statistical details on inflatables made by these and other manufacturers in the fact grids that follow this section.

AIRE

AIRE, based in Boise, Idaho, has been building inflatable boats since 1989. It uses a system in which a removable PVC bladder is inserted inside a very tough skin of PVC-coated polyester. If you experience a tear, you simply unzip the outer skin and replace the inner bladder.

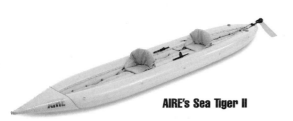

AIRE's Sea Tiger II

The 9-foot, 6-inch Force playboat has a continuous rocker for ease of spinning and surfing. The 32-inch width permits both speed and stability. The cockpit has flotation bags in bow and stern that reduce the

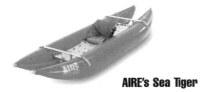

AIRE's Sea Tiger

amount of water that enters the cockpit while improving the ease of rolling. The stern flotation also serves as an adjustable seat back. The 30-pound Force also features a portable three-piece rigid foam floor and center drain holes. Price: $950.

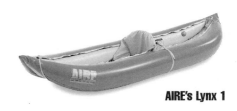

AIRE's Lynx 1

The Cheetah Paddlecat, at 11 feet and 43 pounds, uses a four-tube design that permits a shortened waterline for easy spinning. Increased flotation provides a shallow draft for low-water runs. Price: $950.

The updated version of AIRE's Lynx inflatable has a narrowed front, reducing surface area to increase speed and improve surfing. An extra set of drains was added in front to speed up the self-bailing. The 10-foot, 3-inch Lynx comes with a choice of floors: closed-cell ethafoam or inflatable. The economical rigid-foam floor offers high-performance and dependability, while the inflatable floor is lighter, packs smaller, and is especially good for fly-in or backpacking trips. Price: $950 (foam floor); $1150 (inflatable floor).

The Lynx II is the tandem version of the

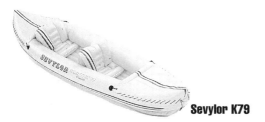

Sevylor K79

Lynx. The greater length (12½ feet) provides increased stability but still lets you paddle solo. Web loops in the floor give lots of seating options so you can paddle tandem or solo in a variety of positions. The Lynx II also comes with the choice of a foam or an inflatable floor. Price: $1050 (foam floor); $1250 (inflatable floor).

The 14-foot, self-bailing Super Lynx features a full-length V-hull for good tracking. Inflatable floor only. Price: $1350.

Jumbo

Jumbo Inflatables, a subsidiary of Zodiac and imported into the United States by Sevylor, offers a complete line of inflatable kayaks.

The Canyon is presented as a light-weight design with lively performance. The self-bailing, buoyant Canyon is 10 feet, 2 inches long, and weighs between 21 and 24 pounds. Two lateral straps give the kayaker precision control over the craft, and an expert can even Eskimo-roll it. Price: $800 (foam floor); $900 (inflatable floor).

The 12-foot, 8-inch Sioux provides a low center of gravity for stability and maneuverability. Its seats convert into backrests at a single tilt. The duck-bill self-bailer rapidly evacuates water from the boat, and a double floor consisting of a removable floor and the boat's bottom protects against abrasion. Weight is 35 pounds. Price: $800.

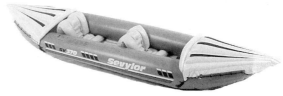

Sevylor SV370

The new wider design of the Tramper SL (31 inches) provides increased stability and interior space over previous models. The Tramper, with a length of 12 feet, 8 inches, has a tubular air floor fitted with stabilizing fins for better tracking. Price: $900.

Catamaran Kayaks

Now inflatable kayaks come in a catamaran design (most people call them "catyaks"). These small catamarans are the ultimate self-bailing boat. Two tubes are held together with a metal frame. Because the open center is wet in whitewater, many boaters add a coated-fabric floor, which allows for greater storage of gear.

Catyaks have a number of advantages. They track well because the tubes rest deeper in the water, and they're extremely stable for the same reason. Best of all, the catyaks break down into small pieces (two tubes and a frame) for easy transportation.

A catyak, however, cannot carry as much weight as an inflatable with a floor (the floor provides additional buoyancy). And some kayakers believe that catamarans are slower in moving current.

Paddling Magazines

To stay informed of the latest developments in kayaking, you might consider subscribing to one or more of these publications:

American Whitewater
American Whitewater Association
P.O. Box 85
Phoenicia, NY 12464
(914) 688–5569

Canoe & Kayak
P.O. Box 3146
Kirkland, WA 98083
(800) 692–2663
(206) 827–6363
Fax (206) 827–1893

Currents
National Organization for River Sports

P.O. Box 6847
Colorado Springs, CO 80904
(719) 473–2466

Paddler
America Canoe Association
7432 Alban Station Boulevard
Suite B-226
Springfield, VA 22150
(703) 451–0141

Sea Kayaker
P.O. Box 17170
Seattle, WA 98107
(206) 789–9536

Manufacturers of Inflatable Kayaks

AIRE
P.O. Box 3412
Boise, ID 83703
(208) 344–7506
Fax (800) 701–2473

B&A Distributing Company
201 SE Oak Street
Portland, OR 97214
(503) 230–0482

Custom Inflatables
P.O. Box 800
Reedsville, WV 26547
(304) 864–3506

Harmon Incept Industries
3347 Highway 8 East #7
Moscow, ID 83843
(208) 882–2884

Hyside Inflatables
P.O. Box Z
Kernville, CA 93238
(760) 376–3723

Innova Recreational Products
180 West Dayton
Suite 202
Edmonds, WA 98020
(425) 776–1171
Fax (425) 778–0115

Jack's Plastic Welding
115 South Main
Aztec, NM 87410
(505) 334–8748
Fax (505) 334–1901

Jumbo Inflatables
6651 East 26th Street
Los Angeles, CA 90040
(213) 727–6013
Fax (213) 726–0481

North American Paddlesports Association
245 North Wauwatosa Road
Mequon, WI 53097
(414) 2432-5228

Northwest River Supplies
2009 South Main
Moscow, ID 83843
(800) 635–5202
(208) 882–2383
Fax (208) 883–4787

Sevylor USA
6651 East 26th Street
Los Angeles, CA 90040
(213) 727–6013
Fax (213) 726–0481

Star Inflatables
232 Banks Road
Travelers Rest, SC 29690
(864) 836–2800
Fax (864) 836–4640

WaterWolf
P.O. Box 169
Telluride, CO 81435
(970) 728–3897
Fax (970) 728–5150

Inflatable Kayaks

The following grids present details on the lineup of inflatable kayaks offered by selected manufacturers. Above are the addresses and phone numbers of these and other manufacturers.

Manufacturer/model	Length (feet)	Width (inches)	Weight (pounds)	Material	Price (dollars)
AIRE (1989)					
Caracal I	10'10"	34	26	PVC-coated polyester	650 (foam floor); 800 (inflatable floor)
Caracal II (tandem)	13'4"	34	33	PVC-coated polyester	750 (foam floor); 900 (inflatable floor)
Cheetah Paddlecat	11'	38	43	PVC-coated polyester	950
Force	9'6"	32	30	PVC-coated polyester	950
Lynx	10'3"	36	28	PVC-coated polyester	950 (foam floor); 1150 (inflatable floor)
Lynx II (tandem)	12'6"	36	43	PVC-coated polyester	1050 (foam floor); 1250 (inflatable floor)
Super Lynx	14'	36	36	PVC-coated polyester	1350
Sea Tiger	16'9"	36	39	PVC-coated polyester	1750
Sea Tiger II (tandem)	19'9"	36	45	polyester/PVC	1850
B & A (1972)					
Momentum Falcon I	10'10"	36	39	Hypalon-coated nylon	950
Momentum Falcon II (tandem)	11'6"	38	46	Hypalon-coated nylon	1050
Momentum Falcon III (tandem)	12'6"	37	51	Hypalon-coated nylon	1100
Riken Cherokee	9'6"	35	43	Hypalon-coated nylon	1300
Riken Commanche	10'9"	38	46	Hypalon-coated nylon	1400
Riken Seminole I	9'6"	35	44	Hypalon-coated nylon	1350
Riken Seminole II (tandem)	10'10"	38	51	Hypalon-coated nylon	1350
Custom Inflatables (1989)					
Thrillseeker PVC-coated	9'2"	36	36	PVC-coated polyester	1250
Thrillseeker II (tandem)	14'6"	36	38	PVC-coated polyester	1400
Thrillkat	10'	37	18	PVC-coated polyester	600
Thrillkat II (tandem)	13'8"	37	24	PVC-coated polyester	800
Harmon Incept (1992)					
Sage	9'6"	24	26	PVC-coated polyester	1300
K-345	11'2"	37	32	PVC-coated polyester	1350
K37D (tandem)	12'7"	42	45	PVC-coated polyester	1500
K38D	12'6"	37	39	PVC-coated polyester	1450
Hyside (1982)					
Padillac I	9'4"	40	39	Hypalon-coated nylon	1100
Padillac II (tandem)	11'9"	40	49	Hypalon-coated nylon	1400
Innova (1992)					
Helios 340 Touring	11'2"	30	25	PVC-coated nylon	600
Helios 380 Touring (tandem)	12'6"	30	29	PVC-coated nylon	650
Helios 380EX Touring	12'6"	30	33	PVC-coated polyester	800
Junior	8'	25	12	PVC-coated nylon	300
Sunny Touring	12'9"	33	33	PVC-coated polyester	700
Vabond	12'6"	38	37	PVC-coated polyester	950

Manufacturer/model	Length (feet)	Width (inches)	Weight (pounds)	Material	Price (dollars)
Jack's Plastic Welding (1982)					
Jack's Yack I	10'6"	37	43	PVC-coated polyester	1100
Jack's Yack II (tandem)	13'	37	40	PVC-coated polyester	1200
Pack Cat I	10'6"	34	24	PVC-coated polyester	1000
Pack Cat II (tandem)	14'	34	32	PVC-coated polyester	1350
Northwest (1972)					
MaverIK I	9'9"	36	35	Hypalon-coated nylon	950
MaverIK II (tandem)	12'3"	36	46	Hypalon-coated nylon	1100
Sevylor (1948)					
K79 Tahiti HF	10'7"	31	25	PVC	150
K79 Tahiti Classic	10'7"	31	25	PVC	150
K79V Vista Kayak	10'7"	31	25	PVC	150
SV370 Sevymarine Kayak	12'	34	29	PVC-coated polyester	600
Star Inflatables (1989)					
K100 Lighting I	10'7"	35	35	PVC-coated nylon	850
K200 Lightning II (tandem)	12'	35	42	PVC-coated nylon	1000
WaterWolf (1988)					
James White	11'6"	24	25	polyurethane-coated nylon	750
Paddlecat Cargo	9'10"	38	34	polyurethane-coated nylon	1300
Paddlecat2 Cargo	13'	38	60	polyurethane-coated nylon	1650
Paddlecat	9'10"	38	25	polyurethane-coated nylon	900
Paddlecat2	13'	38	39	polyurethane-coated nylon	1100
Rapidcat	9'10"	34	20	polyurethane-coated nylon	1000
Rapidcat2	13'	34	20	polyurethane-coated nylon	1200

(Year in parentheses is year the company began making boats)

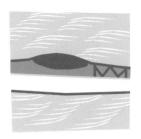

Chapter 13
Build-your-own Kayaks

There's an alternative to buying a manufactured kayak: you can build your own. Several companies offer do-it-yourself kits, consisting of marine-grade mahogany plywood that you cover with fiberglass cloth and epoxy resin. It's possible to end up with a fine touring kayak at a fraction of the cost of a manufactured boat.

The time it takes to complete the boat obviously varies with the particular model and your woodworking skills. Eighty to one hundred hours is not unusual for a first-time builder. The so-called "stitch-and-glue" construction used for these kayaks has revolutionized the building of wooden boats. This technique produces a boat that is stronger and lighter than one built with traditional methods of woodworking. The job goes much faster and requires far less skill. No forms or frames are required.

Here's a brief description of how stitch-and-glue boats are assembled:

- The precut hull panels are aligned to their full length.
- The hull panels are joined with short twists of copper wire. The hull is glued together with epoxy resin and fiberglass, and the inside of the boat is coated with resin.
- The copper wires are snipped off, a layer of fiberglass cloth is placed over the hull, and epoxy is rolled on to form a strong outer layer.
- The deck beams and bulkheads are glued into the boat.
- The deck is glued and tacked down to the sides. The excess plywood is trimmed, and the deck is coated with epoxy resin.
- The cockpit coaming, seat, and backrest are glued on. After a light sanding, the boat is ready for painting or varnishing. Finally, the foot braces and deck rigging are installed.

Instructional Video

The video *Build Your Own Sea Kayak* is available from Great River Outfitters, 4180 Elizabeth Lake Road, Waterford, MI 48328; (248) 683–4770.

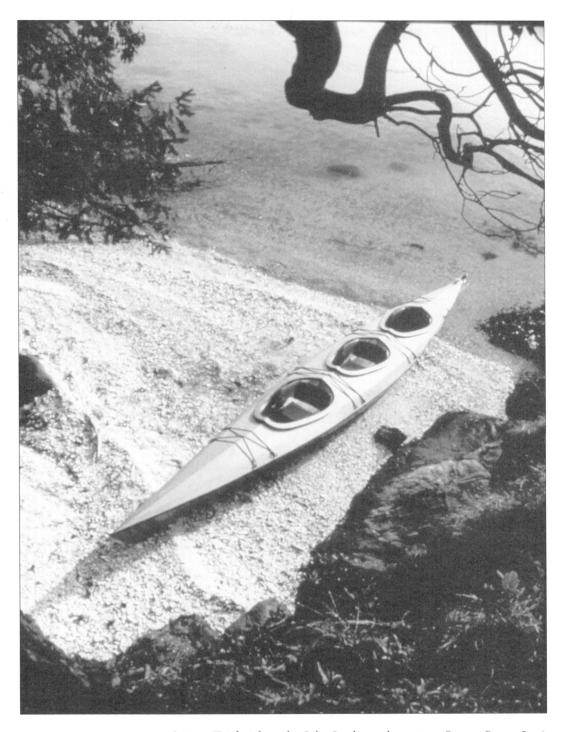

Osprey Triple (photo by John Lockwood, courtesy Pygmy Boats, Inc.)

Build-your-own Kayaks

The following grid presents details on the lineup of kayak kits offered by Chesapeake Light Craft and Pygmy Boats. All models are built of marine-grade mahogany plywood covered with fiberglass cloth and epoxy resin.

Manufacturer/model	Length (feet)	Width (inches)	Weight (pounds)	Keel	Bottom	Sides	Price (dollars)
Chesapeake (1990)							
Cape Charles Series	13', 15'6", 17', 18'	22-25	30-39*	moderate rocker	shallow V	flared	500-600*
Chesapeake Series	15'9", 17',18'	23-24	42-46*	straight with rise at ends	shallow V	flared	650-700*
Mill Creek Series	13', 16'5"	29-33	36-55*	straight	flat	flared	650-700*
Patuxent Series	17'6", 19'6"	21-22	34-40*	straight	shallow V	flared	600-650*
Pocomoke	19'10"	28	52	straight	rounded V	flared	700
Severn	14'6"	26	25	straight with rise at ends	rounded V	flared	450
Tred Avon Double	21'	30	62	straight with rise at ends	shallow V	flared	700
Tred Avon Triple	21'	30	62	straight with rise at ends	shallow V	flared	750
West River Series	16'2", 16'4"	23-24	38	straight	rounded V	flared	650
Yare	16'3"	24	62	straight with rise at ends	rounded V	flared	500
Pygmy (1987)							
Coho Expedition	17'6"	23	39	moderate rocker	rounded V	flared	700
Goldeneye Series	10', 13', 15'8"	17½, 22, 24	14-40*	straight with rise at ends	rounded V	flared	500-650*
Osprey Series	15'8", 17'6", 20'	22, 24, 30	38-61*	straight with rise at ends or moderate rocker	rounded V	flared	700-1000*
Queen Charlotte Series	17', 17'6", 19'	24, 25½	38-45*	straight with rise at ends	shallow V	flared	600-650*

(Year in parentheses is year the company began offering kayak kits)

* Depending on model, material, or options

Good Reads: Building Your Own Kayak

Several excellent books are available for those who wish to make their own boats. Most of the boats described in these books employ traditional woodworking methods rather than the stitch-and-glue process of the plywood kits.

The Kayak Shop: Three Elegant Wooden Kayaks Anyone Can Build, by Chris Kulczycki (Camden, Maine: Ragged Mountain Press, 1993)

Canoes and Kayaks for the Backyard Builder, by Skip Snaith (Ragged Mountain Press, 1989)

Wood and Canvas Kayak Building, by George Putz (Ragged Mountain Press, 1980)

The Strip-Built Sea Kayak: Three Rugged, Beautiful Sea Kayaks You Can Build, by Nick Schade (Ragged Mountain Press, 1998)

The Aleutian Kayak: Origins, Construction, and Use of the Traditional Seagoing Baidarka, by Wolfgang Brinck (Ragged Mountain Press, 1995)

Baidarka: The Kayak, by George Dyson (Edmonds, Washington: Alaska Northwest Publishing Company, 1986)

Manufacturers

Chesapeake Light Craft
1805 George Avenue
Annapolis, MD 21401
(410) 267–0137
Fax (301) 858–6335

Pygmy Boats
P.O. Box 1529
Port Townsend, WA 98368
(360) 385–6143
Fax (360) 379–9326

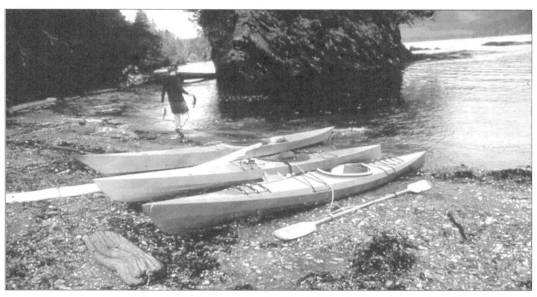

Osprey standard (front), Goldeneye standard (middle), and the Queen Charlotte 19' (rear) (photo by John Lockwood, courtesy Pygmy Boats, Inc.)

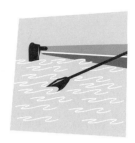

Chapter 14
Paddling Accessories

What accessories do you need before you hit the water? Standard paddling accessories—a life jacket and a spray skirt (and a helmet and flotation bags for whitewater and surf kayakers)—are necessary. The right clothing is also important in paddling to ensure you'll be comfortable. Then there are cartop carriers and camping equipment to consider as well. With the plethora of gear available, only the final selection of what to buy will pose a problem.

Outfitting Your Kayak

A kayak comes from the factory with few amenities. You'll need to customize it to make it more comfortable and more river- or sea-worthy. This customizing includes interior bracing (padding), a back support, a spray skirt to keep water out, and interior flotation bags if better buoyancy is needed.

Hip, Knee, and Thigh Braces (Padding)

Your kayak needs to fit snugly around your hips in order to transfer your body's movements to the boat. You'll lean and execute turns and Eskimo rolls more efficiently with such control. Padding the sides of the seat area with closed-cell foam will give you that custom fit.

Likewise those areas where your knees and thighs come in contact with the kayak should be custom padded. The added comfort and control are remarkable. The only caveat is that if you add braces, you still are able to exit the boat easily if need be. The extra padding for your kayak will cost about $30 to $50.

Back Support

The muscles of the back are actively used in paddling, so good back support is imperative not only for comfort but for effective paddling strokes. Most kayak seats

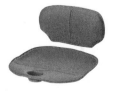

Perception's back and seat pad

have good back supports, but if yours doesn't, it is possible to add a padded backband. Additional back support will cost about $35 to $50.

Flotation Bags

A kayak full of water will sink if it does not have compartments that trap air either

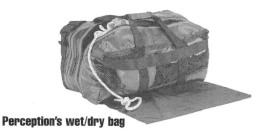

Perception's wet/dry bag

through the use of bulkheads (as used in almost all sea kayaks and most casual touring boats) or flotation bags (as used in most whitewater boats). One flotation bag is usually placed in front of the foot braces and another in the stern behind the seat. For boats with foam pillars, there are "split" bags that fit on either side. To inflate the bags after they are placed inside the kayak, you simply use the long tube attached. Some flotation bags allow storage of gear inside the bag before inflating it. You can purchase flotation bags for $40 to $70.

Spray Skirt

A spray skirt has one basic, but very important, function—to keep water out of the boat. This is important during an Eskimo roll, of course, but is also crucial when you are upright because a dry boat is a warm boat.

Most spray skirts are made from coated nylon or neoprene. Nylon is less expensive, but adequate under most conditions. Neoprene is not only more durable, but warmer (which could be a drawback in warmer climes). Whichever model you choose, make certain it fits snugly around the cockpit rim, but not so tightly that it's difficult to pull it off when you need to exit the boat.

Among the companies that make spray skirts are Harmony, Snap Dragon, Rainbow Designs, Perception, and Wildspray. Spray skirts range in price from $25 to $95.

Other Essentials for the Boat

Before you head out, even for a day trip, you'll also need some other accessories to keep you safe and comfortable, such as:

Hand bilge pump ($10–$30)
Rescue line ($50–$80)
First-aid kit ($20–$50)
Sponge ($5–$10)
Map case ($10)
Waterproof bag ($20–$50)

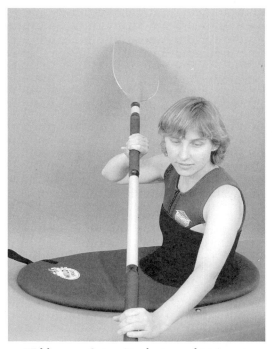

Wildwasser Supra Deck spray skirt (courtesy Prijon/Wildwasser Sport USA)

Life Jackets

No accessory is more important than the life jacket. A number of personal flotation devices, or PFDs as they're called by the U.S. Coast Guard, are now specifically designed for kayakers. Better yet, there are models designed just for whitewater kayakers (which provide greater buoyancy) and for touring kayakers (which are lighter and less restrictive).

Various amounts of flotation are available. For whitewater or large bodies of water, you'll want a high-flotation jacket. For any use, there should be enough buckles and straps to secure the jacket about your body. Most models have pockets and lashing straps for rescue knives and other safety equipment. Kayaking life jackets range in price from $50 to $180.

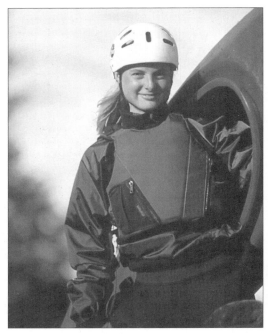

Surfeit side zip PFD (© Phil Deriemer, courtesy Kokatat)

Helmets

For most types of kayaking, and especially whitewater, a helmet is an important piece of safety equipment. As with life jackets, there are many models on the market. The best kayaking helmets are designed some-what like bicycle helmets and have a plastic shell completely lined with foam. The helmet should fit snugly, but not too tightly.

The most popular models are made by Protec, Wildwater, and Prijon. Prices generally range from $40 to $60.

Clothing

Never before have kayakers had such an array of clothing designed just for their needs. New fabrics, insulations, and designs allow a boater to be comfortable in all conditions. The best quality clothing is expensive, but it would be hard to put a price on comfort if you were hypothermic and miles from nowhere.

The general advice is to layer your clothing so you can adjust the amount of clothing you wear as your body heats up or

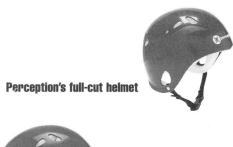

Perception's full-cut helmet

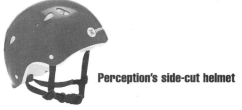

Perception's side-cut helmet

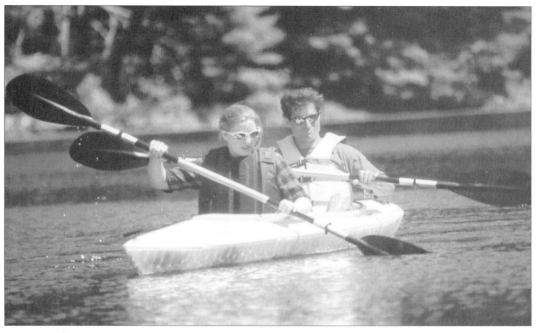

PFDs from Stearns Manufacturing (© Dimaggio/Kalish Water Sports)

cools down. Most kayaking trips involve periods of exertion and rest, which require a boater to remove layers and add clothing, respectively. In cool conditions, you'll want to start with an inner layer of long under-

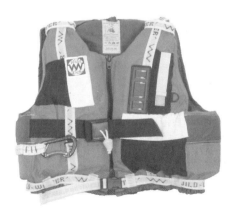

Wildwater Explorer Leader Rescue Lifejacket (courtesy Prijon/Wildwasser Sport USA)

wear and add additional layers of insulation as you need them. When there's a chance of getting wet, add a waterproof shell on top.

Synthetics

The big advantage of today's synthetic fabrics—polyester, polypropylene, fleece, and pile—is their ability to dry quickly. A number of these materials are available in thicker constructions for more warmth. The biggest disadvantage of fleece and pile is that they aren't compact.

Underwear

Polypropylene and polyester underwear work well for kayakers because they don't absorb water. These fabrics are thin (though thicker versions are available for colder or more sedate trips), and thus they don't provide much insulation. But you will be warmer when you are dry.

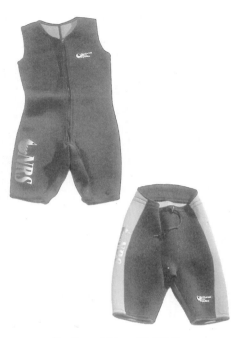

**Northwest River Supplies'
rodeo shorts and little John**

When the temperature drops, you can add additional layers of pile, fleece, or thicker synthetic fill. Goose and duck down are ineffective in wet conditions, because they take days to dry. Wool insulates well even when wet, but it has lost its popularity because it is slow to dry and stretches when wet.

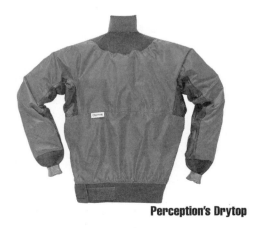

Perception's Drytop

Waterproof Shell

Regardless of what inner layers you wear, you'll need a waterproof outer layer. Kayakers typically use a paddling jacket with tight-fitting closures at wrists, neck, and waist. The market abounds with models containing sophisticated features. Whichever you choose, find one that fits tightly enough to keep you warm and dry, and yet not so tight as to constrict your movement. Paddling pants that feature neoprene ankle cuffs or drysuit seals are available in many styles. Prices generally range from $50 to $115 for paddling jackets and $50 to $75 for paddling pants.

Wet Suits

Neoprene wet suits are used by many paddlers as protection against cold water. The thinner, one-eighth-inch suits are typically chosen. Because sleeved wetsuits hamper upper body mobility during paddling, the most popular model is the sleeveless Farmer John (usually costing $75 to $125). Manufacturers of kayaking wet suits include Patagonia, Northwest River Supplies, and Cascade Outfitters.

Dry Suits

A dry suit made of coated nylon has tight-fitting vinyl seals at neck, wrists, and ankles, which keep you dry, even when doing an Eskimo roll. But a dry suit is cut looser to allow insulation to be worn underneath. As a result, most boaters find dry suits to be more comfortable and versatile than wet suits. Dry suits come in one-piece and two-piece styles. The two-piece suits give you greater versatility when the weather or water warms.

Dry suits are more expensive than wet

suits, and you must be careful to keep the latex seals well lubricated to prolong their life. Prices generally range from $300 to $600 for good quality dry suits. Dry suit tops range from $150 to $350, and dry suit pants range from $100 to $150.

Wet-suit Boots

Wet-suit boots and socks are popular among kayakers because they keep the feet warm in cold water. The sophistication of the newer neoprene shoes is amazing, and some are so rugged and comfortable that it is no longer a problem to wear them for walking considerable distances. Prices range from $25 to $75.

Caps

Remember the adage about keeping the head covered to keep the rest of the body warm? This adage applies to kayakers. In cold weather, most boaters find that their ski caps come in handy.

Gloves

When conditions become frigid, many kayakers use neoprene gloves to keep their hands warm. A drawback of neoprene lies in its elasticity, which over time can tire the muscles of the hand. Other synthetic or fleece gloves are also suitable in cooler conditions or to prevent blisters.

Clothing Makers

A number of companies make clothing designed for kayakers. Patagonia, for example, makes paddling jackets and pants, plus an extensive line of synthetic underwear and insulative garments. Kokatat manufactures a full line of clothing for kayakers. Stohlquist Water Ware offers an array of paddling jackets, as well as a popular line of

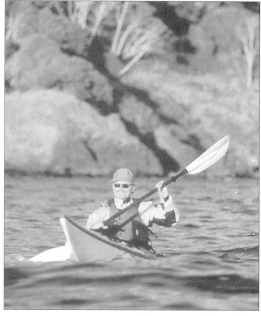

TecTOUR Gore-Tex jacket (© Phil Deriemer, courtesy Kokatat)

dry suits. OS Systems makes an extensive line of dry suits. Northwest River Supplies offers its own brand of wet suits and gloves, as does Cascade Outfitters.

Other manufacturers include Sierra Designs, Rapidstyle, and Palm. The sandals that are ubiquitous among paddlers are made by Teva and Chaco. Among the suppliers of clothing for kayaking are the com-

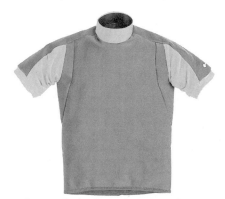

Perception's short sleeve paddling shirt

panies listed at the end of this chapter under Sources of Paddling Accessories.

Cartop Carriers

With the sophisticated car racks available, even the smallest subcompact can transport several kayaks. The accessories for these racks are impressive, and you'll no doubt find the setup that fits your needs perfectly.

One option available with most racks is a set of saddles that conform to the curve of the boat's hull and thus provide a good fit, making it less likely that the rack will deform a plastic kayak. Another option, called a kayak stacker, consists of vertically upright posts fastened to the crossbars. It allows you to stack several kayaks on edge, thereby increasing the capacity of the rack. It adds about $75 to the cost of the rack.

Whatever car rack you use, make sure the boats and gear are securely attached before you hit the highway. Most boaters use either heavy-duty elastic cord or nylon

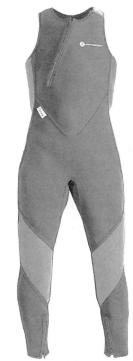

Perception's deluxe farmer john

straps with a strong metal buckle. Even more important, the bow and the stern should be securely fastened to the vehicle's bumpers. Specially made tensioners and hooks are available for this purpose.

Excellent racks, with accessories just for kayaks, are made by Thule, 42 Silvermine Road, Seymour, CT 06483 (800–238–2388) and by Yakima Products, P.O. Box 4899, Arcata, CA 95518 (707–826–8000). Prices generally range from $125 to $250.

Kayak Camping

When a kayaker goes camping, the big problem is storage space in the boat. There just isn't that much room, even in the largest-volume boats. So the search for lightweight, compact camping gear mirrors

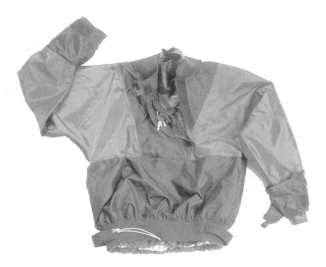

Northwest River Supplies' Plunge Dry-Top

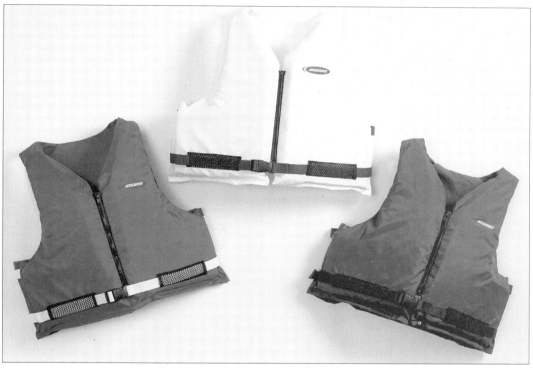

Stearns' personal flotation device 6600 series (courtesy Stearns, Inc.)

that of the backpacker.

Start with good-quality, lightweight camping gear: sleeping bag, camping mattress, and tent appropriate for the climate. And always bring a stove: Campfires can be unreliable, wood may be scarce, and fires are prohibited in some areas. Then there are all the other basics, including such things as cooking equipment, lanterns or headlamps, bug repellent and/or a mesh mosquito jacket, extra clothing, toiletries, ground cloth, and a repair kit.

Checklists: What to Bring Along

The following checklists offer extensive suggestions on items to bring along on kayaking trips. Some of the items are not necessary on every outing, though you may wish to consider carrying them for safety or comfort depending on the destination and conditions. Some items are optional, simply depending on your preference.

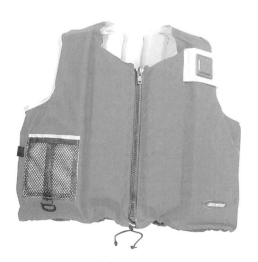

Stearns' 6777 PFD

For more information on items to carry on extended trips, check Chapter 15 for lists of needed safety gear, and Chapter 6 for a list of navigational gear for sea kayaking.

Day Trips
- Paddle
- Personal flotation device
- Helmet
- Throw-rope
- Duct tape/repair kit
- Small first-aid kit
- Sponge/bilge pump
- Lunch
- Water bottle
- Sunscreen
- Clothing suitable for conditions
- Footgear
- Spare clothing
- Waterproof bag
- Rescue gear
- Camera
- Map and guidebook
- Matches and firestarter
- Toilet paper
- Wallet and keys

Overnight Trips
- Paddle, plus a spare
- Personal flotation device
- Helmet
- Throw-rope
- Full repair kit
- Full first-aid kit
- Sponge/bilge pump
- Sunscreen
- Clothing suitable for conditions
- Footgear
- Camp clothing
- Camp shoes
- Wallet and keys
- Carabiner or pulleys for rescues

- Waterproof bags
- Tent or bivy shelter
- Sleeping bag
- Air mattress or pad
- Water containers
- Food
- Cookware and kitchen gear
- Camp stove
- Fuel
- Flashlight
- Map and guidebook
- Navigational equipment/supplies
- Toilet paper
- Plastic trowel
- Insect repellent
- Garbage bags
- Signaling devices
- Camera
- Fishing gear
- Toiletries

Sources of Camping Equipment

The following companies offer catalogs featuring lightweight camping equipment of interest to kayakers.

Campmor
Box 700
Saddle River, NJ 07458
(800) 226–7667

L.L. Bean, Inc.
Freeport, ME 04033
(800) 809–7057
(request Sporting Specialties catalog)

Piragis Northwoods Company
105 North Central Avenue
Ely, MN 55731
(800) 223–6565

Recreational Equipment Inc. (REI)
1700 45th Street East
Sumner, WA 98390
(800) 426–4840

Sources of Paddling Accessories

The following companies offer a wide array of paddling accessories—life jackets, spray skirts, flotation bags, helmets, safety equipment, and so forth. Call for a catalog.

Cascade Outfitters
604 East Forty-fifth Street
Boise, ID 8374
(800) 223–7238
Fax: (208) 322–5016
E-mail: mail@casout.com
Web site: www.casout.com

Four Corners River Sports
P.O. Box 379
Durango, CO 81302
(800) 426–7637
(970) 259–3893
Fax (970) 247–7819
Web site: www.riversport.com

Great River Outfitters
4180 Elizabeth Lake Road
Waterford, MI 48328
(248) 683–4770
(248) 683–0306

Jersey Paddler
Route 88 West
Brick, NJ 08724
(908) 458–5777

Nantahala Outdoor Center Outfitter Store
13077 Highway 19 West

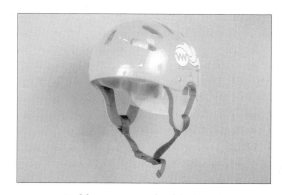

Wildwasser standard helmet (courtesy Prijon/Wildwasser Sport USA)

Bryson City, NC 28713
(800) 367–7521

NOC Outfitter's Store
13077 Highway 19 West
Bryson City, NC 28713
(800) 367–3521
(704) 488–6737
Fax (704) 488–8039
E-mail: storecatalog@noc.com
Web site: www.nocweb.com

Northwest River Supplies
2009 South Main Street
Moscow, ID 83843
(800) 635–5202, (208) 882–2383
Fax (208) 883–4787
E-mail: nrs@moscow.com
Web site: www.nrsweb.com

Piragis Northwoods Company/Boundary Waters Catalog
105 North Central Avenue
Ely, MN 55731
(800) 223–6565
Fax: (218) 365–6220
E-mail: info@piragis.com
Web site: www.piragis.com

Recreational Equipment Inc. (REI)
    1700 45th Street East
    Sumner, WA 98390
    (800) 426–4840
    Web site: www.rei.com

Stohlquist Water Ware
    P.O. Box 3059
    Buena Vista, CO 81211
    (800) 535–3565
    Fax (719) 395–2421
    E-mail: stohlquistwaterware.com
    Web site: http://www.stohlquist.com

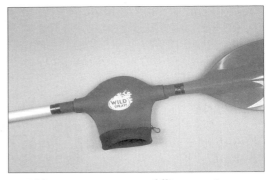

Wildwasser neoprene paddling paw (courtesy
Prijon/Wildwasser Sport USA)

River World
    604 East Forty-fifth Street
    Boise, ID 83714
    (888) 748–3717
    Fax: (208) 322–5016
    Web site: www.riverworld.com

Wyoming River Raiders
    P.O. Box 50490
    300 North Salt Creek Highway
    Casper, WY 82605
    (800) 247–6068
    (307) 235–8624
    Fax: (307) 234–0154
    E-mail: raiders@trib.com
    Web site: www.riverraiders.com

Good Reads: Kayak Camping

Here are a couple of books for people who will be dealing with the challenges of stuffing camping equipment and food into the confines of a kayak:

Kayak Camping, by David Harrison (New York: Hearst Marine Books, 1995)

Kayak Cookery, by Linda Daniel (Birmingham, Alabama: Menasha Ridge Press, 1997)

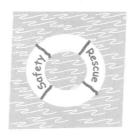

Chapter 15
Safety and Rescue

Kayaking is a safe activity, as long as the boater learns the necessary skills, follows the appropriate safety procedures, and carries the right gear. In this chapter, we'll look at the equipment and techniques that promote safety in sea kayaking and whitewater kayaking, and point to some books and videos that can help paddlers learn more about them. The chapter closes with a discussion of the biggest threat posed to boaters by cold weather and frigid waters, hypothermia, and with recommendations for a kayaking first-aid kit.

Sea Kayaking Safety

The sea kayaker has many devices available to help make ocean touring a safe adventure.

Personal Flotation Device

Make certain you have a good one. ($50–$180) (See the detailed discussion in Chapter 14 on life jackets.)

Bilge Pump

Carry a good handheld bilge pump, and make sure it's securely fastened to the boat. Or get a deck-fitted bilge pump, which provides the most efficient bailing under varied conditions and affords an extra margin of safety, especially for serious deep-water expeditions. (Handheld pump, $10–$25; deck-fitted pump, $75–$150)

Compass

Most boaters find that a good marine compass is indispensable. Many kayaks allow for mounting of a compass on the deck. And don't simply have a compass; also know how to use it. ($25–$100)

Flashing Beacons, Flares and Smoke Devices

If you should get into trouble and need help, you'll need a device to alert others. Today's kayakers can choose from flashing beacons, flares, and smoke devices. Marine flares are available in meteor, parachute, and handheld models, each effective in a certain kind of condition. Select alerting

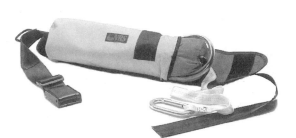

Northwest River Supplies' Pro-Guardian Rescue Kit

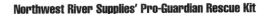

devices that are waterproof or keep them in waterproof containers. (Plan to spend from $25 to $75 on alerting devices.)

Whistle

Some kayakers carry one of the shrill, super-loud whistles for person-to-person alerts. ($5)

Paddle Float

The paddle float, an inflatable bag that fits on the end of a kayak paddle, is used as a stabilizing outrigger to aid a paddler in reentering the boat after a capsize. ($30)

Sponsons

Sponsons are another type of stabilizer. These pontoons inflate with a few puffs of air, stabilizing your kayak sufficiently to allow you to scramble back aboard. The benefit of the sponson system compared with the paddle float is that you have support on both sides of the kayak, and you still have the paddle available for propulsion. ($50–$75)

VHF Radio

A hand-held VHF radio is generally the most effective emergency signaling device (and it has other important uses, too). Marine VHF radios, using very high frequency channels dedicated to marine users, have a range of 5 to 10 miles at sea level. Once the Coast Guard has received your call for help (either directly via their own powerful antennas or indirectly through another vessel), rescue helicopters can home in on your signal as long as you keep pushing the transmit button periodically. ($300–$500)

EPIRB

An Emergency Position Indicating Radio Beacon (EPIRB) is a locator beacon that sends out an electronic call for help on frequencies monitored all over the world. You have to register your EPIRB, so that rescuers know who they're searching for. It doesn't transmit details of your situation, so

---

Good Reads: Safety and Rescue

Kayakers are fortunate in having several excellent books with invaluable information on safety and rescue. (In addition, many paddling schools offer seminars on safety and rescue; see list of schools in Chapter 4.)

River Rescue (third edition), by Les Bechdel and Slim Ray (Boston: Appalachian Mountain Club, 1997)

Whitewater Rescue Manual: New Techniques for Canoeists, Kayakers, and Rafters, by Charles Walbridge and Wayne A. Sundmacher, Sr. (Camden, Maine: Ragged Mountain Press, 1995)

Derek C. Hutchinson's Guide to Expedition Kayaking on Sea and Open Water, by Derek C. Hutchinson (The Globe Pequot Press, 1999)

you can't explain the nature of your emergency. ($225–$800)

GPS

Advances in technology have also brought us Global Positioning System receivers, which are handheld units that use satellites to tell you precisely where you are on the earth. These can be intimidating to use at first, but the peace of mind they afford is worth the effort. ($100–$600)

Personal Towline

When another boat gets into difficulty and needs a tow, you should have a length of rope—usually three-eighths-inch polypropylene—that can be used for that purpose. Jam cleats are commonly installed on boats for this very reason; your hands are free to paddle, and the boat will not twist as much under the stress of towing.

A good towing rig is as important for a sea kayaker as the rescue rope is for a whitewater paddler, and it should be mounted on all kayaks that are used for serious sea journeys. ($50–$75)

Sea Anchor

You may need a sea anchor as a desperate last measure to avoid broaching in high winds and storm-tossed seas. A sea anchor is essentially an underwater parachute that is unfurled of the bow to hold you in position against wind. ($20–$50)

Sea Sock

A sea sock is a large nylon bag that prevents large amounts of water from getting into your kayak. You place the sea sock over the cockpit coaming and insert it inside the boat. Although sea socks should never replace other means of emergency flotation,

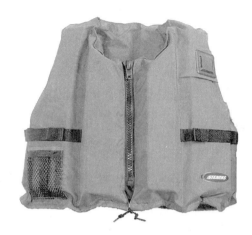

Stearns' 6777 PFD

such as buoyancy bags or bulkheads, they increase the boat's buoyancy and reduce the volume of water entering the boat in a capsize. ($30–$50)

First-Aid Kit

A good first-aid kit is imperative, especially for longer cruises and trips to remote areas. See the end of this chapter for a list of recommended contents for a kayaking first-aid kit. ($20–$50)

Gloves

Blisters will ruin a trip. A good pair of paddling gloves will prevent blisters. ($10–$35)

The whole range of compasses, flares, deck-fitted bilge pumps, VHF radios, and other safety gear needed for sea kayaking

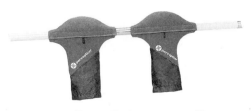

Perception's neoprene mitts

can be found in the catalog from Great River Outfitters, 4180 Elizabeth Lake Road, Waterford, MI 48328; (248) 683–4770.

Sea Kayaking Rescue

Over the years, sea kayakers have developed techniques to help a paddling companion who capsizes. The simplest rescue involves stabilizing the victim's boat to help reentry. This is more difficult than it sounds because of the unwieldy weight of the victim's kayak, which is now filled with water. The potential for injury to the rescuer is great.

Rescue works like this: The victim first needs to place the bow of his or her overturned kayak on the front deck of the rescuer's kayak. As the victim pushes down on the stern, the rescuer lifts the bow to empty the kayak of water. Then the kayak can be turned upright and brought alongside the rescuer's boat.

If getting on board proves impossible for the swimmer (it's much harder than it looks), you can fashion a simple stirrup made of nylon webbing or line to serve as a step for the victim.

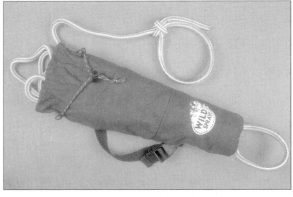

Wildwasser 60-foot safety throwbag (courtesy Prijon/Wildwasser Sport USA)

Check the list of books and videos later in this chapter for sources of detailed information on kayak rescues. The Eskimo roll, a method of self-recovery after a capsize, is used both in sea kayaking and whitewater kayaking, and is described in Chapter 4, paddling technique.

Whitewater Safety

The following are considered essential safety items for whitewater boaters.

Personal Flotation Device. This most indispensable piece of safety equipment must provide sufficient flotation for the water you'll be tackling. ($50–$180)

Helmets. On rocky rivers where overturning is even a slight possibility, helmets provide an important measure of safety. The helmet you choose should be snug, but not so tight that it causes discomfort. The protective internal suspension is usually foam, but cheaper versions have plastic strapping. Whitewater helmets are designed with ear openings so you can hear upcoming rapids and warnings from fellow boaters. ($40–$60)

Throw-rope. For rescue of boaters, the throw ropes made for that purpose are excellent because they float and can be easily tossed. (See the discussion on rescue of others that follows below.) ($50–$80)

Rescue Lines. In the case of rescues, plenty of rope is the key. For boat rescue on difficult rivers, at least fifty feet should be available. Carabiners will also come in handy. ($30–$40)

First-Aid Kit. A good first-aid kit is imperative, especially on long trips to remote areas. ($20–$50)

Sea Touring Safety

According to expert Randel Washburne, there are four rings of defense for sea kayaking safety:

- Avoid Trouble by understanding changeable weather conditions, currents, and tide and by using charts and compasses.

- Survive Rough Seas by bracing, handling beam waves, avoiding a breach, and surfing.

- Recover from a Capsize using the paddle float and techniques of recovery and reentry.

- Signal for Help with pyrotechnics, strobes, or radios.

Washburne says that beginning with the outer ring of defense (Avoid Trouble), the failure of any ring brings into play the need to use the skills associated with the next ring. Weakness in any one skill burdens the rest. The outer rings of defense are the most effective, and the fewer rings you can prevent from being breached, the better your chances of survival. For example, preventing a capsize in rough seas will always be easier than recovering from one in the same conditions.

Repair Kit. The repair kit should include not only repair materials for boats, but also for other equipment. ($20–$40)

River Knives. Most kayakers wear their whitewater safety knife upside down on the life jacket so the knife is readily accessible and easy to pull from the sheath. A serrated edge is more efficient for cutting ropes, and a double-edged knife is better yet. ($25–$60)

Sponge or Bilge Pump. Carry a good bailing device, and make sure it's securely fastened to the boat. ($10–$30)

Whistle. A whistle can be a useful safety device to communicate with other boaters at a distance. ($5)

Gloves. A good pair of paddling gloves can help prevent debilitating blisters. ($10–$35)

Whitewater safety gear can be ordered from the following mail-order companies:

Cascade Outfitters
P.O. Box 209
Springfield, OR 97477
(800) 223–7238
(541) 747–2272

Nantahala Outdoor Center Outfitter Store
13077 Highway 19 West
Bryson City, NC 28713
(800) 367–7521

Northwest River Supplies
2009 South Main Street
Moscow, ID 83843
(800) 635–5205

Whitewater Rescue

It's impossible to overstate the importance of knowing proper whitewater rescue techniques. An excellent reference for learning

Sea Touring Emergency Equipment

Kayaking expert Derek Hutchinson recommends the following equipment for emergencies at sea:

Swiss Army knife
Copper wire
Pliers
Precut stainless steel clips (for joining shock cord elastic)
Cord (for spare bow loop)
Duct tape
Adhesive
Scissors
Sail needle
Heavy-duty thread
Sailor's palm
Waterproof matches
Candles
Bottle of acetone
Epoxy glue
Sharpening stone
Plastic bag containing toilet paper and coins
Waterproof flashlight
Firelighting tablets
Signaling mirror
Fishing line
Fishhooks and weight
Small can opener
Coil of thin, strong line
Heavy-duty polyethylene exposure bag (space blanket)
Patch kit (resin, catalyst, and fiberglass mat)

these techniques is the book *River Rescue* by Les Bechdel and Slim Ray. Rescue experts like Bechdel and Ray advise that you always have safety lines downstream of difficult rapids. The lines will aid in the rescue of boaters who capsize and need assistance getting back on land.

Most safety lines contain 60 to 70 feet of three-eighths-inch polypropylene line in a nylon bag. One end of the line is attached to the bottom of the bag, and the rest of the line is stuffed inside the bag, with the loose end sticking out of the bag.

In a rescue, you grasp or secure the loose end of the line and throw the entire bag to the swimmer. The line will feed out like a spinning reel. Because the swimmer is moving along with the current, you must throw the line downstream of the swimmer's position. Once the swimmer grabs the rescue line, a tremendous pull will be exerted on the line. Be sure you, the rescuer, are well braced.

After the victim grabs the line rope, he or she must turn face up, on the back. The victim should never wrap or tie the rope to his body.

Hypothermia

Hypothermia is a dangerous—and sometimes deadly—lowering of the body's core temperature. Kayakers need to know about this medical condition because a boater can become a victim of hypothermia if exposed to cold conditions long enough. Symptoms typically include fatigue, apathy, forgetfulness, and confusion. Shivering may occur, but not always. Fortunately, hypothermia can largely be prevented by adequate clothing (especially a wet suit or dry suit) and a diet high in sugars and carbohydrates.

This is what happens in hypothermia. The body, thrust into cold, begins to conserve body heat by constricting blood vessels in the arms and legs. As the body attempts to generate heat, shivering usually occurs. Then the body's core temperature starts to drop. As it falls, the person may experience difficulty with speech.

Further drops in temperature bring on symptoms such as muscle stiffness, irrational thinking, amnesia, and unconsciousness. Death can then occur. The most amazing fact about hypothermia is this—in near-freezing water, the time from immer-

Been There, Done That

What more effective way to teach safety at sea than with a collection of real-life stories of kayakers who have gotten into trouble and lived to tell about it? Such a book is now available, and it is gripping. The book is *Sea Kayaker's Deep Trouble: True Stories and Their Lessons from Sea Kayaker Magazine,* by Matt Broze and George Gronseth, and edited by Christopher Cunningham (Camden, Maine: Ragged Mountain Press, 1997).

sion to death can be as short as ten minutes!

Treatment of hypothermia involves warming the victim's body to raise the core temperature. This is done by moving the person out of the wind, replacing wet clothes with dry ones, building a fire nearby, and serving warm beverages (but never alcohol, which actually leads to more loss of heat). It may also be helpful to get inside a sleeping bag with the victim to help warm him or her up.

First-Aid Kit

A good first-aid kit is essential, regardless of the type of paddling you are doing. Be sure that it's adequate for the duration and the location of the trip you're taking, and that it's kept dry and well-stocked.

Sample First-Aid Kit

Assorted adhesive strips (Band-Aids)
Assorted bandages (Ace, triangular, etc.)
Adhesive tape
Gauze roll

Water purification tablets

Aspirin

Seasickness pills

Painkiller

Antiseptic cream

Antibacterial ointment

Antihistamine cream

Sun protection

Snake-bite serum

Scissors

Tweezers

Safety pins

Plastic tubing and airway

First-aid book

Instructional Videos

Paddling guru Kent Ford has produced a couple of instructional videos of interest to both sea kayakers and whitewater boaters: *Performance Sea Kayaking: The Basics and Beyond* and *The Kayakers Edge* (whitewater boating).

They can be ordered from Four Corners River Sports, P.O. Box 379, Durango, CO 81302; (800) 426–7637.

A Final Word

A sourcebook like this is just a beginning. The end is the spirited experiences you will have with the equipment, the techniques, and the books described here. And a glorious end it is. Life, they say, is an adventure only for the adventurous, and kayaking is the perfect medium for pursuing it. Seize the adventure!

A Kayaker's Glossary

Asymmetrical: Hull shape in which the kayak's widest point is either ahead or behind its center.

Beam: The width of a kayak measured at the widest point.

Big water: Rivers with large volume and powerful hydraulics.

Bilge: Transitional area where the hull's bottom turns up into its sides. See chine.

Boulder garden: A river rapids densely strewn with boulders.

Bow: Front of the boat.

Brace: A paddle stroke used to stabilize a tipping kayak. The low brace and high brace are two common techniques.

Breaking wave: In a river, a standing wave that falls upstream.

Broach: To turn sideways to the waves of the sea or to the current of a river; often a dangerous situation.

Broaching sea: Also beam sea; waves and swells coming at the side of the boat.

Bulkhead: Watertight partition that creates a sealed compartment in a kayak; in touring kayaks, this compartment is required for flotation but is also used as a storage area with access via deck hatches.

Casual touring boat: Also called a recreational kayak. A long, high-volume kayak for one or two people, generally used for travel on quiet rivers, sheltered waters, and for low-key touring. Usually somewhat shorter and less expensively built than a sea kayak used for serious touring.

Cfs: Cubic feet per second; a measurement of the volume of water flowing past a given point.

Chine: The transition area between the bottom of the kayak and its sides. See bilge.

Chute: Area where a river's flow is suddenly constricted, compressing and amplifying the current's energy into a narrow tongue of water. See drop, rapids, whitewater.

Coaming: See cockpit.

Cockpit: The opening in the deck of a kayak where the paddler sits. The curved lip around the edge of the cockpit, used to secure the spray skirt, is called the coaming. Keyhole cockpits are elongated to allow easier and safer entry and emergency exits, especially in whitewater.

Cubic feet per second (cfs): A measurement of the volume of a river passing a specified point.

Cushion: See pillow.

Dead reckoning: Distance calculated from time on the water and estimated paddling speed.

Deck: Closed-in area over the bow and stern of a kayak; sheds water.

Depth: Vertical measurement of a kayak from the hull's lowest point to its highest.

Directional stability: The tendency of a kayak to hold its course when under way. See tracking.

Draw stroke: Used to move the boat sideways. Performed by placing the paddle into the water parallel to the boat at an arm's reach away, then pulling boat over to it.

Drop: A steep, sudden vertical change in the riverbed.

Eddy: An area in the river where the current either stops or moves upstream—opposite the main current—usually found below obstructions and on the inside of bends.

Eddy line: Area between main current and eddy current. See eddy.

Ender: A maneuver in which a boat stands up vertically in whitewater; often associated with "playing" in a river.

Entrapment: An often dangerous situation in which a boat and/or paddler is held fast by current and/or an obstacle. See broach, pinned.

Eskimo roll: A self-rescue technique used to right an overturned kayak in the water without leaving the boat.

Feather: To turn the blade of a paddle horizontal to the water.

Ferry: A maneuver used to cross a current with little or no downstream travel. Utilizes the current's force to move boat laterally.

Fiberglass: Glass-fiber cloth impregnated with resin that can be easily formed into hull shapes. This material is relatively cheap, durable, and easy to repair.

Final stability: Also called secondary stability. Describes a boat's resistance to tipping once the boat has been leaned to a point beyond its initial stability.

Flared: A hull shape (viewed in cross-section) that grows increasingly wider as the sides rise from the waterline toward the top edge (the gunwale).

Flat water: Lake water or slow-moving river current with no rapids.

Flotation bags: Inflatable buoyancy bags added to a kayak to ensure that it does not sink when swamped.

Following sea: Waves and swell coming from the stern of a boat.

Grab loops: Short ropes or grab handles threaded through bow and stern of a kayak. Most often used as carrying handles, but also handy for catching swimmers.

Gradient: The steepness of a riverbed over a specified distance, usually per mile.

Hair: Dangerous and difficult whitewater.

Hatch: Access port on front or rear deck of a touring or sea kayak.

Haystack: A large, unstable standing wave in a river.

Hole: See hydraulic.

Hull: The main body of a boat, up to the deck line.

Hull configuration: Shape of the hull or that part of the kayak affected by water, wind, and waves.

Hydraulic: A powerful circulating force of water at the base of a sudden drop.

Hypothermia: The serious medical condition caused by the lowering of body temperature, requiring immediate first aid.

Initial stability: Term used to describe a boat's resistance to leaning or its "tippiness." See secondary stability.

K-1: One-person kayak.

K-2: Two-person kayak.

Keel: A strip or extrusion along the bottom of a boat to prevent sideslipping. Also adds rigidity or structural support to the boat.

Keel line: The longitudinal shape of the kayak's bottom. See hull configuration.

Keeper: A large hole or reversal that can hold a swimmer or a boat for a long time.

Kevlar: A DuPont fiber used as a material for kayak construction. Considerably lighter in weight (30 to 40 percent) than fiberglass, with greater strength and a higher price.

Lay-up: Manner in which layers of fiberglass or Kevlar are applied to make a kayak.

Peel out: The act of leaving an eddy and entering the main current of a river.

Pillow: A cushion of water that forms on the upstream side of rocks or other obstacles.

Pinned: The situation of a boat caught broadside on an obstruction. Most common on steep, shallow rivers. See broach, entrapment.

Playboat: Whitewater playboat.

Playing: A general term for surfing, hole riding, and other maneuvers on a river that go beyond straight downstream paddling.

Polyethylene: Thermoplastic material used in construction of kayaks.

Pool: Relatively quiet area following a rapid or falls in a river.

Pool-and-drop: A river with intermittent rapids followed by long sections of calm water.

Portaging: Traditional term for carrying boats and gear, usually around a rapid or between lakes.

Pry stroke: Turning stroke in which the paddle blade is turned sideways alongside the boat, then pushed outward.

Put-in: The starting place of a paddling trip; where you put your boat in the water. See take-out.

Rapids: Section of a river where the current speeds up and flows turbulently over and around boulders, ledges, shallows, drop-offs, and other features. Also known as

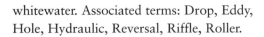

whitewater. Associated terms: Drop, Eddy, Hole, Hydraulic, Reversal, Riffle, Roller.

Reversal: An area of the river where the current turns upstream and revolves back on itself, forming a treacherous current requiring caution; often called hydraulics, stoppers, keepers, curlers, and holes.

Riffle: A shallow section of river characterized by numerous small waves on the surface. Often caused by gravel bars or sand banks.

River-left: On the left side of the river facing downstream.

River-right: On the right side of the river facing downstream.

Rocker: Upward curvature of the keel line from the center toward the ends of a kayak. Lots of rocker means quick, easy turns. See hull configuration, keel line, tracking.

Roller: Large, wide, curling river wave that falls back on itself, usually following a wide rock or obstruction in the riverbed.

Roostertail: A spray of water that explodes when it hits a rock or other obstacle.

Rudder: Steering device (typically foot-controlled) on touring or sea kayaks.

Scout: To examine a rapid from shore.

Scouting: Walking ahead on shore to inspect a rapid, river bend, or a stretch of river.

Sea kayak: Also called a touring kayak. A long, high-volume kayak for one or two people, used for travel on everything from quiet rivers to rough open seas. Most offer considerable stability.

Secondary stability: A hull's tendency to sta-

bilize as it's leaned to one side. See hull configuration, initial stability, final stability.

Sit-on-tops: Kayaks without a cockpit. Sit-on-tops are designed to sit on, not in.

Skeg: Fixed rudder.

Sneak: To take the "easy" route through a rapid.

Sneak route: An easier or safer alternative route around a rapid.

Spray skirt: The "skirt" worn by boaters on decked kayaks to seal the cockpit; usually made of neoprene or nylon.

Squirt boat: An extremely low-volume whitewater kayak designed for play in the underwater currents of a river.

Standing wave: A high river wave caused by deflection of water.

Stern: Back end of a boat.

Stopper: A hole or breaking wave on a river capable of stopping or flipping boats.

Surf: Large breaking waves along a coastline or tidal area. Also a technique for riding large waves on a river or the ocean.

Surf kayak: Kayaks designed for surfing on ocean waves. See surf ski and wave ski.

Surf ski: A type of surf kayak. Short, and featuring a blunt nose, it is derived from the surfboard.

Sweep stroke: Used to turn the boat by reaching out and ahead, then making a stroke in a wide arc.

Sweeper: Fallen trees or brush that lie in the path of the current.

Symmetrical: Hull shape where the kayak's

widest point is at its center. See asymmetrical.

Tail wave: Standing wave that forms at the base of a rapid.

Take-out: The ending point of a paddling trip; where you take your boat from the water. See put-in.

Tandem: Two-person kayak.

Technical: A river with many obstacles that requires constant maneuvering of the currents below the surface as well as on it; for advanced whitewater kayakers only.

Throw bag (throw rope): Rescue device consisting of a rope coiled inside a nylon bag.

Tongue: The smooth V of fast water found at the head of rapids, usually indicating the deepest and least obstructed channel.

Touring kayak: Also called a sea kayak. A long, high-volume kayak for one or two people, used for travel on everything from quiet rivers to rough open seas. Most offer considerable stability.

Tracking: The ability of a boat to hold a straight course due to its design. See directional stability.

Trim: A trim boat is level, side-to-side and end-to-end. Achieved by shifting the load or position of the paddlers.

Tumblehome: A hull with sides that curve inward toward the gunwales. See waterline.

Volume: Used to describe overall capacity of a given hull shape.

Waterline: The position of water along the hull of a boat.

Wave ski: A type of surf kayak; a hard-shelled, foam-filled water craft designed primarily for ocean surfing. The paddler sits on the boat, rather than inside an enclosed cockpit.

Wave train: A series of standing waves in a river.

Whitewater: Turbulent, heavily aerated water caused by its flowing around or over obstacles in the current. See hydraulic, rapids.

Whitewater playboat: A durable and highly maneuverable kayak designed for playing in rapids.

Wrapping: The partial submersion that occurs when a boat's upstream side becomes lodged underwater against a boulder.

Organizations and Clubs

Conservation Organizations

America Canoe Association
7432 Alban Station Road., Suite B-226
Springfield, VA 22150
(703) 451–0141

American Rivers
80l Pennsylvania Avenue SE, Suite 400
Washington, D.C. 20003
(202) 547–6900

American Whitewater Affiliation
136 Thirteenth Street SE
Washington, D.C. 20003
(202) 546–3766

Friends of the River
909 Twelfth Street, Suite 207
Sacramento, CA 95814
(916) 442–3155

National Organization for River Sports
P.O. Box 6847
Colorado Springs, CO 80904
(719) 473–2466

The River Conservation Fund
323 Pennsylvania Avenue NE
Washington, D.C. 20003
(202) 547–6900

United States Canoe Association
606 Ross Street
Middletown, OH 45044
(513) 422–3739

Paddling Clubs

Alabama
Birmingham Canoe Club
P.O. Box 951
Birmingham, AL 35201

Alaska
Juneau Kayak Club
P.O. Box 021865
Juneau, AK 99802

Knik Kanoers & Kayakers
P.O. Box 242861
Anchorage, AK 99524

Arizona
Cochise County Paddle Club
P.O. Drawer T
Bisbee, AZ 85603

Desert Paddling Association
620 East 19th Street
Suite 110
Tucson, AZ 05719

Southern Arizona Paddlers Club
P.O. Box 41927
Tucson, AZ 85717

Arkansas
Arkansas Canoe Club
P.O. Box 1843
Little Rock, AR 72203

California
American River Paddlers
Courtright Road
Lotus, CA 95651

Bay Area Sea Kayakers
P.O. Box 1003
San Rafael, CA 94901

California Kayak Friends
14252 Culver Drive, #A-199
Irvine, CA 92714

California National Canoe Club
Box 1686
Clovis, CA 93613

CSUS Aquatic Center
1901 Hazel Avenue
Rancho Cordova, CA 95670

Environmental Traveling Companions
Landmark Building C
Fort Mason Center
San Francisco, CA 94123

Gold Country Paddlers
637 Hovey Way
Roseville, CA 95678

Hui 0 Hawaii of Sacramento
9242 Cherry Avenue
Orangeville, CA 95662

Kern River Alliance
P.O. Box 294
Kernville, CA 93238

Loma Prieta Paddlers
525 Bonnie View Court
Morgan Hill, CA 95037

Marin Canoe Club
810 ldylberry Road
San Rafael, CA 94903

Miramar Beach Kayak Club
Number One Mirada Road
Half Moon Bay, CA 94019

Popular Outdoor Sport Trips
675 Surrey Lane
Oakland, CA 94605

River City Paddlers
3236 Fitzgerald Road
Rancho Cordova, CA 95742

San Diego Paddling Club
1829 Chalcedony Street
San Diego, CA 92109

San Francisco Sea Kayakers
229 Courtright Road
San Rafael, CA 94901

Santa Cruz Kayak Club
P.O. Box 7228
Santa Cruz, CA 95061

Sequoia Paddling Club
P.O. Box 1164
Windsor, CA 95492

Shasta Paddlers
2515 Park Marina Drive, #104
Redding, CA 96001

Six Rivers Paddling Club
2269 Fickle Hill Road
Arcata , CA 95521

Slackwater Yacht Club
837 Gate 6 Road
Sausalito, CA 94985

Western Sea Kayakers
P.O. Box 59436
San Jose, CA 95159

Western Waters Canoe Club
25252 Terrace Grove Road
Los Galsos, CA 95030

Colorado
Adventure Whitewater Club
1550 North Avenue
Grand Junction, CO 81501

Beartooth Paddlers Society
300 Vine Street
Denver, CO 80206

Colorado Rocky Mountain School
1493 County Road 106
Carbondale, CO 81623

Colorado Whitewater Association
P.O. Box 4315
Englewood, CO 80155

Pikes Peak Whitewater Club
533 North Wasatch Avenue
Colorado Springs, CO 80903

Rocky Mountain Canoe Club
P.O. Box 280284
Lakewood, CO 80228

Rocky Mountain Sea Kayak Club
P.O. Box 100643
Denver, CO 80210

Water Club
P.O. Box 3131
Grand Junction, CO 81502

Connecticut
Columbia Canoe Club
41 Pine Woods Lane
Mansfield Center, CT 06250

Connecticut Canoe Racing Association
153 Chester Street
East Hartford, CT 06108

Conn-Yak
18 Pleasant Street
Burlington, CT 06013

Farmington River Watershed Association
749 Hopmeadow Street
Simsbury, CT 06070

Housatonic Area Canoe & Kayak Squad
104 Kent Road
Cornwall Bridge, CT 06754

Nordkapp Owners Club of North America
47 Argyle Avenue
West Hartford, CT 06107

Sheepshead Canoe Club
7 Lilac Lane
Norwalk, CT 06851

Florida
Apalachee Canoe Club
P.O. Box 4027
Tallahassee, FL 32315

Biscayne Kayakers
5800 Commerce Lane South
Miami, FL 33143

Coconut Kayakers
P.O. Box 3646
Tequesta, FL 33469

Florida Canoe & Kayak Association
P.O. Box 20892
West Palm Beach, FL 33416

Florida Competition Paddlers Association
1725 Georgia Avenue NE
St. Petersburg, FL 33703

Florida Sea Kayaking Association
626 45th Avenue South
St. Petersburg, FL 33705-4418

Florida Sport Paddling Club
276 Spring Run Circle
Longwood, FL 32779

Palm Beach Pack & Paddle Club
P.O. Box 16041
West Palm Beach, FL 33416

Seminole Canoe & Kayak Club
4619 Ortega Farms Circle
Jacksonville, FL 32210

Space Coast Paddlers
P.O. Box 360193
Melbourne, FL 32936

West Florida Canoe Club
P.O. Box 17203
Pensacola, FL 32522

Georgia
Atlanta Whitewater Club
P.O. Box 33
Clarkston, GA 30021

Central Georgia River Runners
P.O. Box 6563
Macon, GA 31208

Georgia Canoeing Association
P.O. Box 7023
Atlanta, GA 30357

Hawaii
Hawaii Canoe/Kayak Team
333 Awini Way
Honolulu, HI 96825

Hawaii Island Kayak Club
74-425 Keal a Kehe Parkway
Kailua-Kona, HI 96740

Hawaiian Sailing Canoe Association
419A Atkinson Drive, #404
Honolulu, HI 96814

Hui Nalu Canoe Club
6077 Summer Street
Honolulu, HI 96821

Hui W'a Kaukahi
c/o Go Bananas
732 Kapahulu Avenue
Honolulu, HI 96816

Kanaka Ikaika Kayak Club
1001 Bishop Street, #2600
Honolulu, HI 96813

Kanaka Ikaika Racing Club
P.O. Box 438
Koneohe, HI 96744

Kihei Canoe Club
P.O. Box 1131
Kihei, Maui, HI 96753

Maui Kayak Club
5211-D Kupele Street
Lahaina, HI 96761

Waikiki Surf Club
791 Sunset Avenue
Honolulu, HI 96816

Idaho
Idaho River Sports Canoe Club
1521 North Thirteenth Street
Boise, ID 83702

Illinois
Abbott Labs Canoe Club
D-41J Building R-13
North Chicago, IL 60064

Chicago Area Sea Kayaker Association
P.O. Box 440
Naperville, IL 60566

Chicago Whitewater Association
2837 Meadow Lane
Schaumburg, IL 50193

Mackinaw Canoe Club
R 1, Box 314
Maroa, IL 61756

Prairie Slate Canoeists
839 Stratford Lane
Downers Grove, IL 60516

St. Charles Canoe Club
13 Circle Drive West
Montgomery, IL 60538

Saukenuk Paddlers Canoe & Kayak Club
P.O. Box 1038
Moline, IL 61265

Indiana
Hoosier Canoe Club
12330 East 131st Street
Noblesville, IN 46060

Ohio Valley Whitewater Club
219 South Welworth
Evansville, IN 47714

Wildcat Canoe Club
P.O. Box 6232
Kokomo, IN 46904

Iowa
Midwest River Expeditions
P.O. Box 3408
Dubuque, IA 52004

Kansas
Kansas Canoe Association
Box 2885
Wichita, KS 67201

Kentucky
Viking Canoe Club
P.O. Box 32263
Louisville, KY 40232

Louisiana
Bayou Haystackers Canoe Club
10525 Tams Drive
Baton Rouge, LA 70815

Boundary Waters Adventure Association
P.O. Box 1565
Leesville, LA 71446

Maine
Maine Canoe/Kayak Racing Organization
RFD 2, Box 268
Orrington, ME 04474

Penobscot Paddle & Chowder Society
1115 North Main Street
Brewer, ME 04412

Maryland
Blue Ridge Voyagers
13102 Brahms Terrace
Silver Spring, MD 20904

Canoe Cruisers Association
P.O. Box 15747
Chevy Chase, MD 20825

Greater Baltimore Canoe Club
P.O. Box 1841
Ellicott City, MD 21041

Mid-Atlantic Canoe Club
14048 Vista Drive, #308
Laurel, MD 20707

Monocacy Canoe Club
P.O. Box 1083
Frederick, MD 21702

Tantallon International Sea Kayaking Association
12308 Loch Circle
Fort Washington, MD 20744

Massachusetts
Appalachian Mountain Club
5 Joy Street
Boston, MA 02108

Boston Sea Kayak Club
15 Waldron Court
Marblehead, MA 01945

Cape Cod Blazing Paddles
Cape Cod Community College
West Barnstable, MA 02668

Martha's Vineyard Oar & Paddle
P.O. Box 840
West Tisbury, MA 02575

Westfield River Canoe Club
Igell Road
Chester, MA 01011

Michigan
Great Lakes Sea Kayaking Club
3721 Shallow Brook
Bloomfield Hills, MI 48302

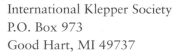

International Klepper Society
P.O. Box 973
Good Hart, MI 49737

Lansing Oar and Paddle Club
P.O. Box 26254
Lansing, MI 48909

Negwegon Kayak Club
218 West Bay Street
East Tawas, MI 48703

West Michigan Coastal Kayakers Association
P.O. Box 1706
Frankfort, MI 49635

Minnesota
Cascaders
P.O. Box 580061
Minneapolis, MN 55458

Minnesota Canoe Association
Box 13567
Dinkytown Station
Minneapolis, MN 55414

Twin Cities Sea Kayaking Association
P.O. Box 581792
Minneapolis, MN 55458

Missouri
Missouri Whitewater Association
325 DeBalviere, #131
St. Louis, MO 63112

Montana
Beartooth Paddlers Society
P.O. Box 20432
Billings, MT 59104

New Hampshire
Merrimack Valley Paddlers
32 Titan Lane
Greenville, NH 03048

New Jersey
Appalachian Mountain Club
64 Lupine Way
Stirling, NJ 07980

Extreme Whitewater
P.O. Box 1841
Rahway, NJ 07065

Garden State Canoe Club
142 Church Road
Millington, NJ 07946

Hackensack River Canoe Club
P.O. Box 369
Bogota, NJ 07603

Hunterdon County Canoe Club
1020 Route 31
Lebanon, NJ 08833

Inwood Canoe Club
238 Union Avenue
Rutherford, NJ 07070

Mohawk Canoe Club
194-A Sawmill Road
Lebanon, NJ 08833

Monoco Canoe Club
304 Elton Adelphia Road
Freehold, NJ 07728

National Canoe Safety Patrol
37 Westview Drive
North Bergen, NJ 07047

North Hudson Academy
P.O. Box 390
North Bergen, NJ 07047

Outdoor Club of South Jersey
109 Worthman Avenue
Bellmawr, NJ 08031

Paddling Bares
P.O. Box 22
Milltown, NJ 08850

Wanda Canoe Club
P.O. Box 723
Ridgefield Park, NJ 07660

New Mexico
Adobe Whitewater Club of New Mexico
P.O. Box 3835
Albuquerque, NM 87190

New York
Adirondack Mountain Club
47 Thorpe Crescent
Rochester, NY 14616

Adirondack Paddlers
P.O. Box 653
Saranac Lake, NY 12983

American Whitewater Affiliation
P.O. Box 85
Phoenicia, NY 12464

Champaign Canoeing
c/o Ann LeClair
Brayton Park
Ossining, NY 10562

Downtown Boat Club
241 West Broadway
New York, NY 10013

Empire Canoe Club
105 Johnson Town Road
Sloatsburg, NY 10974

Greenpoint Canoe and Kayak Club
143 Angent Avenue
Brooklyn, NY 11222

Hilltop Hoppers Canoe/Kayak Club
P.O. Box 47
Rensselerville, NY 12147

Housatonic Area Canoe & Kayak Squad
12 Boltis Street
Mt. Kisco, NY 10549

Inwood Canoe Club
P.O. Box 94
Inwood Station, NY 10034

Ka-Na-Wa-Ke Canoe Club
Old State Road RR #1
Box 77D
Marrisville, NY 13408

Kayak & Canoe Club of New York
P.O. Box 329
Phoenicia, NY 12464

Metropolitan Association of Sea Kayakers
195 Prince Street, Basement
New York, NY 10012

Metropolitan Canoe and Kayak Club
P.O. Box 021868
Brooklyn, NY 11202

Midtown West Parents Association
345 Eighth Avenue, #17F
New York, NY 10001

Nissequogue River Canoe Club
P.O. Box 2302
Huntington, NY 11743

Paumanok Paddlers
18 Stuart Court
Hampton Bays, NY 11946

Rinky Dink Canoe Club
1751 67th Street
Brooklyn, NY 11204

St. Lawrence Valley Paddlers
P.O. Box 616
Canton, NY 13617

Sebago Canoe Club
1751 67th Street, #B-8
Brooklyn, NY 11204

Staten Island Canoe Club
37 Wyona Avenue
Staten Island, NY 10314

Sugar Island Canoe & Kayak Club
14 Deer Meadow Road
Warwick, NY 10990

Touring Kayak Club
205 Beach Street
City Island, Bronx, NY 10464

Wooden Canoe Heritage Association
P.O. Box 226
Blue Mountain Lake, NY 12812

Yonkers Canoe Club
12 Autumn Circle
Yonkers, NY 10703

Zoar Valley Paddling Club
1195 Cain Road
Angola, NY 14006

North Carolina
Carolina Canoe Club
P.O. Box 12932
Raleigh, NC 27605

Nantahala Racing Club
P.O. Box 134
Almond, NC 28708

Triad River Runners
P.O. Box 24094
Winston-Salem, NC 27114

Western Carolina Paddlers
7 Garden Terrace
Asheville, NC 28804

Wilderness Center Alumni Club
2711 Spring Bridge Trail
Greensboro, NC 27410

Ohio
Dayton Canoe Club
1020 Riverside Drive
Dayton, OH 45405

Keel Haulers Canoe Club
1649 Allen Drive
Westlake, OH 44145

Outdoor Adventure Club
P.O. Box 402
Dayton, OH 45404

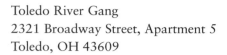
Toledo River Gang
2321 Broadway Street, Apartment 5
Toledo, OH 43609

Oregon
Cascade Canoe Club
1595 Cottage Street NE
Salem, OR 97303

Lower Columbia Canoe Club
11231 NE Davis Street
Portland, OR 97220

Northwest Whitewater Association
P.O. Box 19008
Portland, OR 99202

Oregon Kayak & Canoe Club
P.O. Box 692
Portland, OR 97207

Portland Kayak & Canoe Team
2463 NW Quimby Street
Portland, OR 97210

River Ramblers Canoe & Kayak Club
917 Norman Avenue NE
Salem, OR 97301

South Oregon Association of Kayakers
1951 Roberts Road
Medford, OR 97504

Willamette Kayak & Canoe Club
P.O. Box 1002
Corvallis, OR 97339

Pennsylvania
Canoe Club of Greater Harrisburg
RD 1, Box 421
Middleburg, PA 17842

Conewago Canoe Club
P.O. Box 138
Bigierville, PA 17307

Lancaster Canoe Club
133 Belvedere Avenue
Pomeroy, PA 19367

Lehigh Valley Canoe Club
P.O. Box 4353
Bethlehem, PA 18018

Philadelphia Canoe Club
4900 Ridge Avenue
Philadelphia, PA 19128

Three Rivers Paddling Club
811 Smokey Wood Drive
Pittsburgh, PA 15218

Western Pennsylvania Paddle Sport Association
110 Thornwood Lane
Slippery Rock, PA 16057

Wilmington Trail Club
323 North Shore Lane
Landenburg, PA 19350

Rhode Island
Rhode Island Canoe Association
70 Scott Street
Pawtucket, RI 02860

South Carolina
Foothills Paddling Club
P.O. Box 6331
Greenville, SC 29606

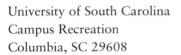

University of South Carolina
Campus Recreation
Columbia, SC 29608

Tennessee
Eastman Recreation Club
400 South Wilcox Drive
Kingsport, TN 37662

Tennessee Scenic Rivers Association
P.O. Box 24094
Nashville, TN 37215

Tennessee Valley Canoe Club
P.O. Box 11125
Chattanooga, TN 37401

University of Tennessee Canoe & Hiking
    Club
2106 Andy Holt Avenue
Knoxville, TN 37996

Texas
Aggieland Paddle Club
7988 Drummer Circle
College Station, TX 77845

Alamo City Rivermen
2622 Moss Bluff
San Antonio, TX 78234

Austin Paddling Club
P.O. Box 14211
Austin, TX 78761

Bayou City Whitewater Club
P.O. Box 980782
Houston, TX 77098

Dallas Downriver Club
P.O. Box 595128
Dallas, TX 75359

Hill Country Paddlers
P.O. Box 2301
Kerrville, TX 78029

Houston Canoe Club
P.O. Box 925516
Houston, TX 77292

North Texas River Runners
215 Lakeshore Drive
Waxahatchie, TX 75165

Texas Canoe Racing Association
2610 Choctaw Trail
Austin, TX 78745

Texas Seatouring Kayak Club
P.O. Box 27281
Houston, TX 77227

Utah
Utah Whitewater Club
P.O. Box 520183
Salt Lake City, UT 84152-0183

Vermont
Club/Team Adventure
P.O. Box 184
Woodstock, VT 05091

Virginia
Association of North Atlantic Kayakers
34 East Queens Way
Hampton, VA 23669

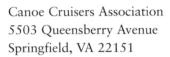

Canoe Cruisers Association
5503 Queensberry Avenue
Springfield, VA 22151

Coastal Canoeists
P.O. Box 566
Richmond, VA 23204

Float Fishermen of Virginia
P.O. Box 1750
Roanoke, VA 24008

Mid-Atlantic Paddlers Association
P.O. Box 1346
Gloucester Point, VA 23062

Smith River Valley Canoe Club
15 Cleveland Avenue, #8
Martinsville, VA 24112

Washington Canoe Club
1906 Windmill Lane
Alexandria, VA 22307

Washington
Northwest Whitewater Association
P.O. Box 4941
Spokane, WA 99202

Paddle Trails Canoe Club
P.O. Box 24932
Seattle, WA 98124

Puget Sound Paddle Club
P.O. Box 22
Puyallup, WA 98371

Southwest Washington Canoe Club
505 Williams-Finney Road
Kelso, WA 98626

Washington Kayak Club
3048 62nd Ave NW
Seattle, WA 98116

Washington Recreational River Runners
P.O. Box 25048
Seattle, WA 98125

West Virginia
Mason-Dixon Canoe Cruisers
Route 1, Box 169-31
Falling Waters, WV 25419

West Virginia Wildwater Association
P.O. Box 8413
South Charleston, WV 25303

Wisconsin
Green Bay Paddlers United
1741 Westfield Avenue
Green Say, WI 54303

Hoofers Outing Club
800 Langdon Street
Madison, WI 53703

Wausau Kayak/Canoe Corp.
915 Fifth Street
Wausau, WI 54401

Canada
Alliance of British Columbia Sea Kayak
    Guides
221 Ferntree Place
Nanaimo, British Columbia V9R 5M1

Barris Canoe Club
P.O. Box 23
Barrio, Ontario L4M 1G0

Cowichan Kayak and Canoe Club
5086 MeLay Road, RR 3
Duncan, British Columbia V9L 2X1

Great Lakes Sea Kayaking Association
P.O. Box 22082
45 Overlea Boulevard
Toronto, Ontario M4H IN9

Missinipe Big Water Club
Box 1110
La Ronge, Saskatchewan, S0J 1L0

Ocean Kayak Association of British Co-
lumbia
P.O. Box 1574
Victoria, British Columbia V8W 2X7

Ocean Kayak Association of British Columbia
Sidney Chapter
2420 Amelia Avenue
Sidney, British Columbia V8I 2J3

Ottawa Sea Kayaking Club
5968 Byron Avenue
Ottawa, Ontario K2A 0J3

Sea Kayak Association of British Columbia
Box 751, Postal Station A
Vancouver, British Columbia V6C 2NC

Victoria Sea Kayaker's Network
752 Victoria Avenue
Victoria, British Columbia V8S 4N3

Index

BRACE YOURSELF

If you are one of the 1.4 million people who kayak, our carefully researched guides written by the top names in the business are must-reads. Whether you are a novice or expert, a surf, sea, or whitewater kayaker, The Globe Pequot Press has books that discuss it all, from choosing equipment to mastering acrobatics.

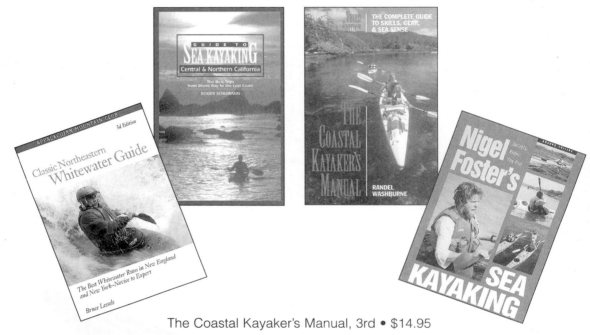

The Coastal Kayaker's Manual, 3rd • $14.95

Guide to Sea Kayaking: Southern Florida • $15.95

Derek C. Hutchinson's Basic Book of Sea Kayaking • $7.95

Guide to Sea Kayaking: Central and Northern California • $15.95

Classic Northeastern Whitewater Guide, 3rd • $19.95

The Complete Book of Sea Kayaking, 4th • $19.95

Nigel Foster's Sea Kayaking, 2nd • $14.95

IT'S GOING TO BE A WILD RIDE

To place an order or request a catalog:
Call 9-5 EST: 800-243-0495 • Fax: 800-820-2329 • www.globe-pequot.com
The Globe Pequot Press, P.O. Box 833, Old Saybrook, CT 06475